# TABLE OF CONTENTS

WW Instant pot Breakfast recipes ............... 6
- Italian Creamy Chicken Pasta Recipe ................. 6
- Italian Pulled Pork Ragu ................. 7
- Weight Watchers Breakfast Casserole ................. 9
- Homemade Onion Soup Mix ................. 10
- Homemade Sausage Recipe ................. 11
- Fajita Breakfast Casserole ................. 12
- Starbucks Sous Vide Egg Bites ................. 14
- Banana French Toast ................. 15
- Weight Watcher Pancakes ................. 17
- Pumpkin Puree Recipe ................. 18
- Instant Pot Oatmeal ................. 19
- Cheesy Egg Bake ................. 20
- Instant Pot Cinnamon Apples ................. 21
- Instant Pot Mashed Potatoes ................. 22
- Candied Sweet Potatoes ................. 23
- Applesauce Recipe ................. 24
- Weight Watchers Apple Cake ................. 25
- Un-stuffed Cabbage Bowls ................. 26
- Beef Drip Sandwiches ................. 27
- Spaghetti with Meat Sauce ................. 28
- Sausage Cabbage Bowl with Quinoa ................. 29
- Pork Carnitas (Mexican Pulled Pork) ................. 31

WW Instant pot Launch recipes ................. 33
- Instant Pot Potato Leek Soup ................. 33
- Instant Pot Chipotle Chicken Tacos ................. 34
- Stuffed Pepper Soup Recipe ................. 36

- Burrito Bowl ..................................................................................................... 37
- Chicken Cacciatore ............................................................................................ 39
- Instant Pot Shrimp Recipes ............................................................................... 40
- Instant Pot Buffalo Chicken Dip ........................................................................ 41
- Buffalo Chicken Wings ...................................................................................... 42
- Instant Pot Chicken Tikka Masala with Cauliflower and Peas ........................... 44
- Macaroni and Cheese ....................................................................................... 46
- Buffalo Chicken Wings ...................................................................................... 47
- Instant Pot Jambalaya ....................................................................................... 49
- Instant Pot BBQ Chicken Bowls ......................................................................... 51
- Spanish Rice with Chicken ................................................................................ 52
- Spicy Beef and Broccoli Stir Fry ........................................................................ 54
- Instant Pot Beef Stew ....................................................................................... 56
- Homemade Baked Beans Recipe ...................................................................... 57
- Mexican Spiced Instant Pot Cauliflower Soup .................................................. 58
- Instant Pot Spicy Tomato Sauce ....................................................................... 59
- Instant Pot Honey Garlic Chicken ..................................................................... 60
- Instant Pot Jerk Chicken Soup .......................................................................... 61
- Protein Packed Chicken Stew ........................................................................... 62
- Split Pea Soup with Ham .................................................................................. 64
- Spaghetti Squash Pad Thai (Low Carb) ............................................................. 65
- Chickpea Sweet Potato Stew ............................................................................ 67
- Barbacoa Beef (Instant Pot) .............................................................................. 68
- Turkey Meatball Stroganoff .............................................................................. 69

WW Instant pot DINNER recipes .............................................................................. 71
- Garlicky Cuban Pork .......................................................................................... 71
- Healthy Tuscan Chicken Pasta .......................................................................... 72
- Shredded Mexican Chicken .............................................................................. 74
- BBQ Pulled Pork Recipe .................................................................................... 75

# Fresh & Fast WW Program Cookbook 2024

Mouthwatering Collection of Quick & Easy to Follow, Delicious WW Recipes for Living and Eating Well Everyday

By

Sonya Mc. Reeves

Copyright © **Sonya Mc. Reeves** 2024

All rights reserved. No part of this publication maybe reproduced, stored or transmitted in any form or by any means, electronic, mechanical, photocopying, recording, scanning, or otherwise without written permission from the author. It is illegal to copy this book, post it to a website, or distribute it by any other means without permission.

**Sonya Mc. Reeves** moral right to be identified as the author of this work.

| | |
|---|---|
| Instant Pot Goulash | 76 |
| Roasted Chicken Breast & Vegetables | 77 |
| Instant Pot Vegetable Noodle Soup | 78 |
| Vegan Instant Pot Mushroom Soup | 79 |
| Healthy Beef Stew | 83 |
| Instant Pot Vegetable Soup | 85 |
| Cheesy Turkey Burger Macaroni | 86 |
| Spicy Asian Chicken Soup | 87 |
| Chicken Enchilada Soup | 88 |
| Skinny Steak Soup | 89 |
| Instant Pot Beef and Barley Stew | 90 |
| Beef and Tomato Stew | 92 |
| Chicken Curry Recipe with Potatoes | 93 |
| Chicken and Dumplings | 94 |
| Chicken and Rice Recipe | 96 |
| Buffalo Chicken Lettuce Wraps | 97 |
| Instant Pot Chicken Soup | 98 |
| Brussels Sprouts with Bacon and Garlic | 100 |
| Meatloaf Mashed Potatoes | 101 |
| Mushroom Barley Soup | 103 |
| Light Stuffed Pepper Soup | 104 |
| Boneless Pork Chops Recipe | 105 |

# WW INSTANT POT BREAKFAST RECIPES

## Italian Creamy Chicken Pasta Recipe

Prep time: 10 mins //Cook time: 15 mins
Serves: 8 // **Points Values: 6**

Makes 8 Servings 1½ cup per serving 8 SmartPoints per serving

### Ingredients

- 1 pound boneless skinless chicken breast, cubed & 16oz box penne pasta
- 2 cups chicken stock (or water) & 2 Roma tomatoes, diced
- ½ red onion, diced & 1 cup mushrooms, diced
- 2 cloves garlic, minced (can use equivalent garlic powder if you prefer) & 2 teaspoons Italian seasonings
- 1 cup low-fat part-skim mozzarella cheese, shredded & ½ cup fat-free cream cheese

### Instructions

- At first Add all ingredients to Instant Pot liner, except for cheeses.
- Next Mix well so that pasta is covered in liquid and everything is well combined.
- Then Place lid and set to seal.
- After that Set to high pressure (manual) for 9 minutes. Once done, allow to NPR (natural pressure release) for 5 minutes.
- Once pressure has released, remove the lid and stir in cheeses until well combined and melted.

- Finally Serve with additional Parmesan or parsley as desired.

**Nutritional Facts** Makes 8 servings (1 1/2 cup per serving)

## Italian Pulled Pork Ragu

Total Time: varies / Servings : 10, Serving Size: 1/2 cup sauce

**Points Values: 1**

### Ingredients:

- 18 oz pork tenderloin & 1 teaspoon kosher salt
- black pepper, to taste & 1 tsp olive oil
- 5 cloves garlic, smashed with the side of a knife & 1 (28 oz can) crushed tomatoes (I love Tuttorosso)
- 1 small jar roasted red peppers, drained (7 oz jar) & 2 sprigs fresh thyme
- 2 bay leaves & 1 tbsp chopped fresh parsley, divided

### Instructions:

- Season pork with salt and pepper. Press saute button to warm, add oil and garlic and saute until golden brown, 1 to 1 1/2 minutes; remove with a slotted spoon.
- Add pork and brown about 2 minutes on each side.
- Add the remaining ingredients and garlic, reserving half of the parsley.
- Cook high pressure 45 minutes. Natural release, remove bay leaves, shred the pork with 2 forks and top with remaining parsley.
- Serve over your favorite pasta.

**Nutrition Facts Per Serving** Calories: 93 calories / Total Fat: 1.5g /Saturated Fat: g /Cholesterol: 33mg

# Weight Watchers Breakfast Casserole

Prep Time 5 mins // Cook Time 15 mins
Servings 4 // **Points Values: 2**

## Ingredients

- 6 eggs & 6 pieces center cut bacon cooked and crumbled
- 1 cup fat-free cheddar cheese shredded & 1/2 red onion diced
- 1/2 bell peppers diced & 1 teaspoon salt
- 1 teaspoon black pepper , 1/2 teaspoon garlic powder & 1 cup water

## Instructions

- At first In a large bowl, whisk together eggs, salt, black pepper, and garlic powder until well combined.
- Next Mix in bacon, cheese, onion, and peppers until well covered.
- Then Pour into already sprayed casserole dish (I use a small ceramic dish that is safe for oven use)
- After that Pour 1 cup water into the bottom of the Instant Pot Liner
- Create an aluminum foil sling, or use a trivet in the bottom of the liner. Place bowl into the Instant Pot.
- Place lid on Instant Pot and set to seal.
- Choose the manual setting and set to 13 minutes.
- Finally When cooking cycle has completed, allow to NPR (natural pressure release) for 2 minutes. Release remaining pressure and using silicone mitts remove the bowl from the Instant Pot liner.

**Nutrition Facts Per Serving** Calories 162 , Calories from Fat 72 , Total Fat 8g 12% , Saturated Fat 3g 15% , Cholesterol 252mg 84% , Sodium 878mg 37% , Potassium 161mg 5% , Total Carbohydrates 3g

## Homemade Onion Soup Mix

Prep Time: 5 mins // **Points Values: 10**

*Ingredients:*

- ¾ C onion chopped or minced & 3 t parsley
- 2 t onion powder & 1 t turmeric
- ½ t kosher salt
- ½ t ground black pepper & ½ t celery seed

*Instructions*

- First Stir ingredients to mix and Next store in airtight container.
- Then About 1/3 cup equals one packet of store bought onion soup mix.

**Nutrition Facts Per Serving** Calories: 78kcal , Carbohydrates: 17g ,Protein: 2g

# Homemade Sausage Recipe

Prep Time 10 mins // Cook Time 5 mins
Servings: 4 // **Points Values:13**

## Ingredients:

- 1 pound ground turkey or chicken & 1 tsp. cinnamon
- 1 tsp nutmeg & 1/2 tsp salt
- 1/2 green apple chopped small , 1/4 C bone broth & 2 T coconut oil if frying

## Instructions

- At first Put meat, apple, broth, and spices into a mixing bowl.
- Next Mix the ingredients together with your hands.
- Then Form into 12 small patties.
- After that Heat coconut oil in large pan and add sausage patties to hot oil.
- Cook for about 5 minutes, flipping half way.
- Finally You can also bake these in the oven - it's less messy!

**Nutritional Facts Per Serving** Calories: 206kcal, Carbohydrates: 4g, Protein: 27g , Fat: 9g , Saturated Fat: 6g //Cholesterol: 62mg

# Fajita Breakfast Casserole

Prep Time 10 mins // Cook Time 2 mins
Servings: 2 // **Points Values: 2**

## *Ingredients*

- 1/2 cup onion sliced & 1 1/2 cup sliced bell peppers green, red, and orange
- 1 tbsp. olive oil & 4 eggs
- A sprinkle of salt and pepper & For optional garnish: cilantro avocado, and limes

## *Instructions*

- At first Turn the Instant Pot to sauté, add the olive and allow it to heat up. Toss in the garlic, onions, and bell peppers to sauté them. Sauté for about 5 minutes until the edges of the onions and bell peppers start to brown like fajitas.
- Next Turn off the Instant Pot and transfer the bell peppers and onions to a round oven safe pan that will fit inside. I used a 2-quart soufflé pan, but any oven safe dish would work.
- Then Gently crack four eggs and place them on top of the peppers so that the yolk is intact. Sprinkle with salt and pepper then cover with foil. Use a large piece of foil folded into thirds to make a sling to lower and remove the dish from the Instant Pot.
- After that Place the trivet at the bottom of the Instant Pot insert and add 1 cup of water. Gentle lower the dish to sit on top of the trivet. Lock the lid into place and close the pressure valve to sealing. Cook on high pressure for 2 minutes using the manual function. Release pressure using the quick release function.

- Finally Remove the pan from the Instant Pot. Top with avocados, cilantro, and sliced limes. Perfect with a side of whole wheat toast.

# Starbucks Sous Vide Egg Bites

Prep Time 10 mins // Cook Time 18 mins
Servings : 4 // **Points Values:5**

## Ingredients
- 4 Large Eggs & 4 strips bacon (Pork or Turkey)
- 3/4 cup Favorite Cheese & 1/2 cup Cottage Cheese
- 1/4 cup Heavy Cream , 1/2 tsp Salt & Optional: Dash of Hot Sauce

## Instructions
- At first Put 1 cup of water in the bottom of your Instant Pot followed by the trivet that came with your pot.
- Next Cook the bacon utilizing your favorite method to cook bacon. Crumble and evenly distribute into 4 mason jars.
- Then Add the eggs, cheese, cottage cheese, cream and salt to the blender and blend until smooth (about 15 seconds).
- After that Add a dash of hot sauce if desired and blend for a few more seconds.
- Spritz the mason jars with spray oil (no need if using silicon molds)
- Divvy the egg mixture evenly into 4 mason jars.
- Cover each mason jar loosely with foil and place gently in the Instant Pot.
- Place the cover on the Instant Pot and select "Steam" and set to 8 Minutes.
- NPR (natural pressure release) for 10 minutes and then quick release (QR) the rest.
- Carefully remove the egg bites from the Instant Pot and let cool down for a few minutes.
- Finally Enjoy immediately or refrigerate for up to a week!

**Nutrition Facts Per Serving** 170 calories, 7g of fat, 13g of carbs

# Banana French Toast

Prep Time 15 mins//Cook Time 30 mins
Servings 6 // **Points Values:12**

## Ingredients

- 6 slices french bread cut into 3/4 inch cubes & 4 bananas sliced
- 2 tablespoons brown sugar & 1/4 cup cream cheese
- 3 eggs & 1/4 cup milk
- 1 tablespoon white sugar & 1 teaspoon vanilla extract
- 1/2 teaspoon ground cinnamon & 2 tablespoons butter chilled and sliced
- 1/4 cup pecans chopped & Pure maple syrup optional

## Instructions

- At first Slice french bread into cubes.
- Next Grease a 1 1/2 QT round baking dish or cake pan for the 8 qt Instant Pot. If you have a smaller pressure cooking pot, use a baking dish that will fit inside of the pot.
- Then Add a layer of bread to the bowl.
- After that Layer one sliced banana over the bread, then sprinkle one tablespoon of brown sugar over the bananas.
- In a microwave, melt the cream cheese 30-45 seconds until it's creamy enough to spread. Cover the bananas and bread with cream cheese.
- Add the rest of the bread to the bowl and layer one more sliced banana over the bread.
- Sprinkle one tablespoon of brown sugar over the bananas and half of the pecans over the top.
- Place sliced butter pieces over the bread as the top layer.

- In a mixing bowl, beat the eggs with a whisk. Whisk milk, white sugar, vanilla, and cinnamon into egg mixture.
- Pour egg mixture over the bread, making sure to coat the bread well.
- Pour 3/4 cup water into the pressure cooker pot and place a trivet or pot lifter in the bottom of the pot. If you don't have a trivet to lift the pan out of the hot pressure cooker, make a sling out of of a large foil strip.
- Center the pan on the trivet or foil strip and lower it into the pressure cooker.
- Lock the lid in place. Select High Pressure and set the timer for 25 minutes. If using an Instant Pot, select the porridge button, then add 5 minutes to the cook time.
- When timer goes off, turn off the pressure cooker and turn the steam release valve to "venting" to release the pressure. Keep french toast pan in pressure cooker to warm for 5 minutes before removing lid. After 5 minutes and the pressure valve has dropped, remove lid and remove dish from pressure cooking pot.
- Finally Let set for another 5 minutes, then top with sliced bananas, nuts and maple syrup before serving.

# Weight Watcher Pancakes

Prep Time 10 mins // Cook Time 10 mins
Servings: 14 pancakes // **Points Values:1**

## *Ingredients*

- 2 over-ripe bananas mashed & 2 egg whites
- 1 cup of fat-free plain greek yogurt & 1/2 cup of fat-free milk
- 1 teaspoon of pure vanilla extract & 1 cup of all-purpose flour
- 2 teaspoons of baking powder & 1/2 teaspoon of cinnamon

## *Instructions*

- At first Preheat a nonstick electric skillet to 325 degrees.
- Next In a medium sized bowl, combine mashed bananas, egg whites, greek yogurt, milk and vanilla extract. Then Whisk until well combines.
- After that In a larger bowl, combine flour, baking powder and cinnamon and whisk.
- In the next step Stir wet ingredient into dry ingredients.
- Finally Pour 1/4 cup of batter onto hot skillet and cook until golden brown.

**Nutrition Facts Per Serving** Calories 40, Sodium 58mg, Total Carbohydrates 10g

## Pumpkin Puree Recipe

Prep Time 5 mins // Cook Time 18 mins
**Points Values:0**

### Ingredients
- 1 small sugar (pie) pumpkin (about 2 - 3 pounds)

### Instructions

- At first Add steamer rack to InstantPot Pressure cooker.
- Next Add 1 cup water to pressure cooker.
- Then Place pumpkin on rack inside pressure cooker and make sure the lid seals. If the stem is too tall, trim stem until lid seals properly.
- After that Seal pressure cooker cover and cook on HIGH pressure for 13 minutes.
- In the next step Your InstantPot pressure cooker will take some time to build up the pressure and temperature inside.
- After the 13 minute cooking time finishes, allow your InstantPot to release the pressure naturally for at least 10 minutes. Then if you want to release it manually, go ahead. Or, just let it completely release on its own.
- Once the pressure is released, remove the cover and carefully lift out the rack, being careful not to drop the pumpkin which will be very hot.
- Place pumpkin on a cutting board and cut in half.
- Scoop out seeds and pumpkin goop. Feel free to rinse and drain pumpkin seeds for later use.
- Peel cooked pumpkin from the skin and add to Vitamix or other high-powered blender or food processor. Process to desired consistency.
- Finally Scoop out fresh pumpkin puree and store in airtight container in the refrigerator.

**Nutrition Facts Per Serving** Amount Per Serving (1/2 cup), Calories 38 Calories from Fat 3 , Total Carbohydrates 9.1g 3% ,Dietary Fiber 3.3g 13% ,Protein 1.2g

## Instant Pot Oatmeal

Prep Time 5 mins//Cook Time 5 mins
Servings 4 // **Points Values:3**

### *Ingredients*

- 1 c oats use steel oats if you like a more turgid oatmeal & 2 1/2 c water
- 1 c apple skinned and diced , 2 tbsp brown sugar , 3 tbsp butter & pinch cinnamon , raisins optional

### *Instructions*

- At first Put Instant Pot or pressure cooker on manual high pressure.
- Next Add butter and allow to melt. Turn Instant Pot off...important step to avoid "burn" message from showing up.
- Then Add water, oats, brown sugar, apples, cinnamon and raisins if desired. Stir
- Finally Put lid on and close steam valve, set to manual high pressure for 5 minutes, do a quick release, open and serve.

*Nutrition Facts Per Serving* Amount Per Serving (6 oz) /Calories 192 Calories from Fat 90/ Total Fat 10g 15% / Saturated Fat 5g 25% /Cholesterol 22mg 7%

# Cheesy Egg Bake

Prep Time: 5 mins // Cook Time: 20 mins
Servings: 4 // **Points Values:4**

## *Ingredients*

- 6 slices bacon, chopped & 2 cups frozen hash browns
- 6 eggs, ¼ cup milk & ½ cup shredded cheddar cheese
- 1 teaspoon kosher salt, ½ teaspoon pepper & optional add-ins: onion, red pepper, spinach, mushrooms, green onions

## *Instructions*

- First Chop up bacon into small pieces then saute in pressure cooker until crispy.
- Next Add in any extra veggies that you would like and saute until tender, about 3 minutes.
- Then Add in frozen hash browns and stir until slightly thawed, about two minutes.
- After that Grease a heat proof container that will fit into your Pressure Cooker. I used a round metal bowl.
- Whisk together eggs, milk, shredded cheese, and salt and pepper in a separate bowl and then add bacon and veggie mixture to the eggs.
- Pour the egg mixture into your greased, heat proof container.
- Pour 1 ½ cups of water into your pressure cooker and set trivet inside. Place heat proof bowl with egg mixture on top of trivet.
- Lock lid and set to high pressure for 20 minutes with a quick release at the end.
- Loosen edges then dump out onto large plate.
- Finally Serve with green onions and extra shredded cheese!

# Instant Pot Cinnamon Apples

Prep Time: 5 mins// Cook Time: 2 mins
Servings: 4-6 // **Points Values:0**

## Ingredients

- 3 apples (we like gala)
- 1 heaping tsp cinnamon
- 1 heaping tsp maple syrup

## Instructions

- At first Peel, core, and slice the apples. (I use this tool that does it all at once!).
- Next Combine apples, cinnamon, and maple syrup in the Instant Pot. Pour in 1/4 cup water. Stir quickly to coat the apples.
- Then Cook on high pressure for 2 minutes. Quick release. Serve immediately or remove lid and keep warm until you're ready (up to an hour).

**Nutrition Facts Per Serving** Serving Size: 4oz / Calories Per Serving: 42 / Cholesterol 0mg

## Instant Pot Mashed Potatoes

Total Time:20 mins// Prep Time:10 mins
Servings : 06, Serving Size: 3/4 cup // **Points Values: 5**

### *Ingredients:*

- 2 pounds peeled Russet potatoes, quartered & 3 cups water
- 1/2 teaspoon kosher salt & 1/3 cup low-fat 1% buttermilk
- 1/4 cup light sour cream (I prefer Breakstone's) & 2 tablespoons whipped butter
- 1 teaspoon kosher salt , fresh black pepper, to taste & chopped chives or parsley, for garnish

### *Instructions:*

- At first Add potatoes to the instant pot and pour enough water to just cover, season with salt.
- Next Cover and cook on high pressure 10 minutes, quick release to check the potatoes are soft. They are done when a sharp knife can easily be inserted through the potato.
- Then Drain and reserve 1/2 cup of the water, add the butter, sour cream and buttermilk, salt and black pepper and mash with a potato masher.
- Adjust salt to taste and keep on warm until ready to serve. It's best to eat right away, but if you're eating them later and the potatoes get dry, add the reserved water to loosen them.
- Finally Serve garnished with chopped chives or parsley.

***Nutrition Facts Per Serving*** Calories: 142 calories / Total Fat: 4g /Saturated Fat: 2.5g /Cholesterol: 11.5mg

| Candied Sweet Potatoes |
|---|

Prep Time 5 mins // Cook Time 28 mins
Servings 8 // **Points Values: 4**

## *Ingredients*

- 4 cups diced sweet potatoes approximately 2 large & 1/2 cup orange juice
- 1 tablespoon blackstrap molasses & 1 tablespoon cinnamon
- 1/4 cup sugar & 1 teaspoon vanilla

## *Instructions*

- At first Prepare Instant Pot liner with 1 cup water in bottom and trivet placed.
- Next Prepare Instant Pot safe bowl or casserole dish by spraying with non-stick spray.
- Then Peel and dice sweet potatoes into 1/2"-1" chunks.
- After that Pour into casserole dish and add cinnamon, sugar, molasses, vanilla, and orange juice.
- In the next step Mix until well combined.
- Place into Instant Pot on top of the trivet.
- Place the lid and set to seal.
- Cook on manual pressure for 20 minutes.
- Finally NPR (natural pressure release) for 8 minutes.

***Nutrition Facts Per Serving***, FreeStyle, and Flex Plans, Makes 8 Servings (1/2 cup per serving)

## Applesauce Recipe

Prep Time 15 mins // Cook Time 20 mins
Serves : 8 // **Points Values: 1**

### *Ingredients*

- 5 large Gala apples & 5 Golden Delicious apples
- 2 tbsp pure maple syrup , 1 tsp ground cinnamon & 1/4 cup water

### *Instructions*

- At first Peel and core the apples. Next Thinly slice and cut each slice in quarters.
- Then Place the apples into a large bowl.
- After that Add the maple syrup and cinnamon to the apples. Stir to combine.
- In the next step Pour the water into the bottom of the Instant Pot. Add the apples.
- Put the lid on the Instant Pot, close the steam vent and to HIGH pressure using the manual setting. Decrease the time to 5 minutes.
- Let the steam release naturally for 5 minutes, then carefully use the quick release valve to release the steam.
- Finally Break up any apple chunks with a wooden spoon. Serve or store in the refrigerator.

**Nutrition Facts Per Serving**: Serving Size 1/2 cup / Calories 143.5 cal Calories from fat 0 / Carbohydrate 35.4g / Dietary Fiber 5.9g / Sugars 28.6g /Protein 0.6g

# Weight Watchers Apple Cake

Prep Time 10 mins // Cook Time 30 mins
Servings : 8 // **Points Values: 6**

## *Ingredients*

- 2 cups flour , 1 cup oats & 1/2 cup sugar substitute suitable for baking
- 1/4 teaspoon salt & 1/4 teaspoon baking soda
- 2 teaspoons cinnamon & 1 teaspoon vanilla extract
- 1/2 cup unsweetened applesauce &, 2 cups apples diced & 1/2 cup unsweetened almond milk you can use original or vanilla as long as unsweetened

## *Instructions*

- At first Place the trivet and 1 cup water into Instant Pot liner.
- Next Spray a bowl or dish that fits into your Instant Pot with non-stick spray.
- Then Combine all ingredients in a large mixing bowl and stir until well combined.
- After that Pour into prepared bowl or dish and place onto trivet inside Instant Pot liner.
- Place the Instant Pot lid and set to seal.
- Set to Cake function for 25 minutes. Allow to cook, and when complete, NPR (natural pressure release) for 5 minutes.
- Finally Release remaining pressure, remove and serve.

**Nutrition Facts Per Serving** Calories 275 Calories from Fat 126 / Total Fat 14g / Saturated Fat 11g / Cholesterol 40mg / Sodium 162mg

## Un-stuffed Cabbage Bowls

Total Time: 30 minutes
Makes about 6 cups // **Points Values: 8**

### Ingredients:

- cooking spray & 1 lb 93% lean ground beef
- 1 1/4 teaspoon kosher salt & 1 cup chopped onion
- 1 clove garlic, minced & 1 tablespoon dried marjoram
- black pepper, to taste & 8 ounce can tomato sauce
- 1/2 teaspoon Hungarian paprika & 1 cup less sodium beef broth
- 2 tablespoons raisins, 1 cup cooked brown rice & 1 medium head cabbage, cored and chopped (9 cups)

### Instructions

- At first Press the saute button on the Instant Pot. Next Spray with oil then add the beef and salt, cook breaking the meat up until browned, about 5 minutes. Then Add the onion, garlic, marjoram and black pepper and stir. Add the tomato sauce, paprika, beef broth and raisins, cover and cook high pressure 15 minutes.
- Quick release, finally add the rice and cabbage and cook 3 minutes high pressure. Quick release and serve with additional rice if desired.

**Nutrition Facts Per Serving** Calories: 338 calories / Total Fat: 8g /Saturated Fat: 3g /Cholesterol: 71mg

# Beef Drip Sandwiches

Prep Time: 5 Min// Cook Time: 1 Hrs, 10 Min
Serving Size: 1 sandwich // **Points Values:8**

## *Ingredients*

- 2 lb lean beef eye round roast & 1 onion, chopped
- 1 cup beef broth & 8 oz pepperoncini with juice, jarred
- 1/2 tsp salt & 3 tbsp Italian seasoning
- 8 reduced calorie hamburger rolls & 1 green pepper, sliced
- 1 red pepper, sliced & 1 cup part skim shredded mozzarella cheese

## *Instructions*

- First Add the beef, onion, pepperoncinis, beef broth, salt, and Italian seasoning the Instant Pot (or another pressure cooker). Next Cover and cook on high for 1 hour. Carefully vent the pressure cooker and shred the beef using two forks. For a slow cooker, cook on low for 8 hours.
- Finally Lightly toast each roll in the broiler. Top with beef, thinly sliced peppers, and two tablespoons of cheese. Return to broiler and cook for about one minute until cheese melts.

**Nutrition Facts Per Serving** Serving Size: 1 sandwich/ Calories 290 //Calories from Fat 64 //Cholesterol 75mg

## Spaghetti with Meat Sauce

Total Time:30 mins // Prep Time:5 mins
Servings : 5, Serving Size: scant 1 1/2 cups  // **Points Values: 10**

### Ingredients:
- 1 lb 93% ground turkey & 3/4 teaspoon kosher salt
- 1/4 cup diced onion & 1 clove minced garlic
- 1 jar (25.25 ounces) Delallo Tomato Basil Pomodoro Sauce & 2 cups water
- 8 ounces whole wheat or gluten-free spaghetti, I used Delallo & Grated parmesan cheese, optional for serving

### Instructions:

- At first Press saute on the Instant Pot. When hot add the turkey and salt and cook, breaking up about 3 minutes.
- Next Add the onions, and garlic and cook until softened, 3 to 4 minutes.
- Then Add the Pomodoro sauce, water and spaghetti (broken in half), making sure the liquid covers everything without stirring.
- In the next step Cover and cook on high pressure 9 minutes.
- Finallay Quick release so the pasta doesn't continue cooking, and serve topped with grated cheese if desired!

**Nutrition Facts Per Serving** Calories: 390 calories /Total Fat: 14g /Saturated Fat: g /Cholesterol: 64mg

# Sausage Cabbage Bowl with Quinoa

Prep Time 10 mins // Cook Time 42 mins
Serves 6 // **Points Values: 5**

## *Ingredients*

- 2 tsp olive oil , 1 lb. hot or sweet Italian chicken sausage (raw) & 1 yellow onion, chopped
- 3 garlic cloves , 1 tsp paprika & 1 tsp dried oregano , 3/4 tsp salt
- 1/2 tsp ground pepper & 1 1/4 cup low sodium chicken broth
- 1 cup canned petite diced tomatoes & 1/2 cup dry quinoa
- 1 3/4 lb. cabbage, thinly sliced (about 12 cups) , 1/4 cup minced Italian parsley & Salt and pepper, to taste

## *Instructions*

- First Set Instant Pot to Saute setting. Next Add the olive oil and allow to heat for 30 seconds. Then Add the chicken sausage (squeezed out of casings) and onion, and cook, breaking up the sausage with a wooden spoon, until the sausage is browned, about 5 minutes. Stir in the garlic, paprika, oregano, salt and pepper.
- After that Add the chicken broth and diced tomatoes, and stir to combine.
- In the next step Put the lid on the Instant Pot, close the steam vent and set to HIGH pressure using the manual setting. Decrease the time to 12 minutes. (It will take about 15 minutes for the Instant Pot to reach pressure.)
- Once the time is expired, carefully use the quick release valve (it may sputter a bit) to release the steam.
- Stir in the quinoa and pile the cabbage on top (don't stir it in). Put the lid on the Instant Pot again, close the steam

vent and set to HIGH pressure. Decrease the time to 3 minutes. Release the steam using the quick release valve.
- Finally Stir in the parsley and season to taste. Serve.

**Nutrition Facts Per Serving** Serving Size 1 1/3 cups / Calories 233.5 cal Calories from fat 72 / Total Fat 8.9g /Saturated Fat 2.3g /Cholesterol 55.0mg

# Pork Carnitas (Mexican Pulled Pork)

Total Time: 80 minutes
Servings : 11, Serving Size: 1/2 cup // **Points Values: 3**

## Ingredients:

- 2 1/2 pounds trimmed, boneless pork shoulder blade roast, cut into 4 pieces , 2 teaspoons kosher salt
- black pepper, to taste & 6 cloves garlic, cut into sliver
- 1 1/2 teaspoons cumin & 1/2 teaspoon sazon (I used homemade)
- 1/4 teaspoon dry oregano & 1 cup reduced sodium chicken broth
- 2-3 chipotle peppers in adobo sauce (to taste) & 2 bay leaves
- 1/4 teaspoon dry adobo seasoning (I used Goya) & 1/2 teaspoon garlic powder

## Instructions:

- First Season pork with salt and pepper.
- Next Press saute on the instant pot, spray with oil and brown the pork on all sides for about 5 minutes. Remove from heat and allow to cool.
- Then Using a sharp knife, insert blade into pork about 1-inch deep, and insert the garlic slivers, you'll want to do this all over.
- After that Season pork with cumin, sazon, oregano, adobo and garlic powder all over.
- In the next step Pour chicken broth, add chipotle peppers and stir, add bay leaves and place pork in the Instant Pot, cover and cook using the pressure cooker setting on high pressure for 80 minutes.
- When the pressure releases, shred pork using two forks and combine well with the juices that accumalated at the bottom.

- Finally Remove bay leaves and adjust cumin and add adobo and mix well.

**Nutrition Facts Per Serving** Calories: 160 calories / Total Fat: 7g /Saturated Fat: 3g /Cholesterol: 69mg

## WW INSTANT POT LAUNCH RECIPES

### Instant Pot Potato Leek Soup

Prep Time 10 mins // Cook Time 10 mins // **Points Values: 4**

### Ingredients

- 4 cups low sodium chicken broth & 1 pound peeled and cubed white potatoes (You can use Yukon Gold)
- 1 lb leeks (I used a bag of frozen from Trader Joe's) & 1 teaspoon sea salt
- 1 teaspoon cracked pepper , 1 teaspoon crushed garlic & 1 teaspoon extra virgin olive oil

### Instructions

- First Using the sauté function, add olive oil, sliced leeks and salt and sauté until soft. Next Add the crushed garlic; sauté for 30 seconds and then turn off the sauté function. Allow to cool for 2 minutes.
- After that Add in all remaining ingredients. Place lid on top and lock into place. Be sure to close to your pressure vent. Set to high pressure and cook for 11 minutes.
- Once your IP is done, do a quick pressure release. Pull out your immersion blender, and blend the soup mixture until almost all the lumps of the potatoes have been mixed with the leeks. This creates a yummy creamy texture (as shown in photos). This should take you about 2-3 minutes.
- Finally Serve with parsley on top and enjoy!

**Nutrition Facts Per Serving** Calories: 0 /Total Fat: 0g /Saturated Fat: 0g /Cholesterol: 0mg

# Instant Pot Chipotle Chicken Tacos

Prep Time: 15 mins//Cook Time: 20 mins
Servings: 12 // **Points Values:3**

## *Ingredients*

- 1 medium onion chopped , 1 Tablespoon garlic minced & 1 pound boneless chicken breasts
- 1/2 cup chicken broth & 2 Tablespoons chipotle chiles diced
- 1 teaspoon brown sugar & 1/2 teaspoon garlic powder
- 1 Tablespoon fresh cilantro chopped & 1/2 small lime juiced
- lettuce & 1 medium tomato chopped
- 12 6 inch tortillas & 1/2 cup cheese shredded & olive oil spray

## *Instructions*

- First With the cooker's lid off, spray the olive oil spray and heat to "Saute" until the cooker has heated up. Next Add the onion and garlic and Then cook until the onion is translucent and the garlic is fragrant.
- After that Season the chicken breasts with salt and pepper and place in the Instant Pot and saute until browned. In the next step Add the chicken stock, chilies, brown sugar, cilantro and lime juice. Securely lock the pressure cooker's lid and set to "Manual". Cook at HIGH pressure for 8 minutes.
- Perform a quick release to release the pressure. Open the lid and remove the chicken breasts. Shred the chicken and set it back in the cooker.

- Finally Scoop out 1/2 cup of the chicken mixture onto a tortilla. Add lettuce, tomato and cheese, if desired and serve immediately.

**_Nutrition Facts Per Serving_** Calories: 148kcal /Carbohydrates: 13.1g / Protein: 10.9g /Fat: 5.9g / Saturated Fat: 2.1g / Cholesterol: 29.3mg

# Stuffed Pepper Soup Recipe

This crock pot stuffed pepper soup recipe is an easy weeknight meal! I've also adapted it for the Instant Pot.

Prep Time10 mins // Cook Time8 hrs
Servings: 8 // **Points Values: 3**

## Ingredients

- 1 lb extra lean ground turkey or beef & 1 cup onion, chopped
- 14.5 oz. can diced tomatoes with roasted garlic and onions & 15 oz. can tomato sauce
- 2 cups green and red peppers, chopped (I've added up to four peppers, and it's yummy!) & 3 cups beef broth
- ½ teaspoon basil , 1.5 packets of chili seasoning & 1 cup cooked rice, brown or white

## Instructions

- First Brown ground beef with onion in a skillet over medium heat.
- Next Drain beef and onions and place in instant pot.
- Then Chop peppers, add to instant pot.
- After that Add tomatoes (including juice) and remaining ingredients, except rice – which should be added 1 hour before end of cooking.
- In the next step Cover and cook on low for 6-8 hours.
- Finally Natural pressure release for 10 minutes.

**Notes :** Instant Pot Adaptation: Saute the meat and onion, then add peppers, tomatoes and tomato sauce, broth, and spices. Cook at high pressure 7 minutes, add cooked rice after.

**Nutrition Facts Per Serving** Calories: 247kcal, Carbohydrates: 32.5g, Protein: 15.7g, Fat: 5.2g, Saturated Fat: 1.5g, Cholesterol: 41mg, Sodium: 1015mg, Potassium: 475mg

# Burrito Bowl

This Burrito Bowl recipe is prefect for meal prep day! Cook this Instant Pot Burrito Bowl recipe once and eat all week long!

Prep Time10 mins //Cook Time25 mins

Servings: 6 // **Points Values: 3**

## Ingredients

- 2 frozen chicken breasts & 1/2 cups uncooked brown rice
- 1/2 C dry black beans (not soaked) & 1 - 15 oz can diced tomatoes, no sugar added
- 2 tbsp. Minced garlic & 2 tbsp. Cumin
- 1 tbsp. Onion powder , 2 tbsp. Chili powder & F1.5 cups chicken stock

Toppings for Burrito Bowls:

- Romaine lettuce (green)
- Cheddar cheese (blue)
- Avocado (blue)
- Salsa or pico de gallo (fresh is green)

## Instructions

- First Combine all the ingredients in the Instant Pot. Next Lock the lid into place and seal the pressure valve.
- Then Using the manual mode cook on high pressure for 25 minutes. When done release by turning the pressure valve to open, be sure to use a long spoon or a silicone oven mitt to move the valve.
- After that Open the lid and remove the chicken to shred. I use my mixer to shred chicken–it's SO easy to do! Just make sure to stand right there and watch because the chicken goes from shredded to ground pretty quickly.
- In the next step Add the chicken back into the Instant Pot, stir well.

- Finally Measure and place the romaine lettuce in your bowl. Top with 1/6 of the beans, rice, and shredded chicken. Measure out and sprinkle with cheese, salsa, and avocado if you'd like!

**Nutrition Facts Per Serving** Calories: 464kcal /Carbohydrates: 40g / Protein: 56.3g /Fat: 8.1g / Saturated Fat: 0.4g /Cholesterol: 143mg

# Chicken Cacciatore

Total Time: 35 mins
Servings : 4, Serving Size: 1 thigh with 1/2 cup sauce
**Points Values: 3**

## Ingredients:

- 4 chicken thighs, with the bone, skin removed & kosher salt and fresh pepper to taste
- olive oil spray & 1/2 can (14 oz) crushed tomatoes (Tuttorosso my favorite!)
- 1/2 cup diced onion & 1/4 cup diced red bell pepper
- 1/2 cup diced green bell pepper & 1/2 teaspoon dried oregano
- 1 bay leaf & 2 tablespoons chopped basil or parsley for topping

## Instructions:

- First Season chicken with salt and pepper on both side.
- Next Press saute on the Instant Pot, lightly spray with oil and brown chicken on both sides a few minutes. Set aside.
- Then Spray with a little more oil and add onions and peppers. Sauté until soften and golden, 5 minutes.
- After that Pour tomatoes over the chicken and vegetables, add oregano, bay leaf, salt, and pepper, give it a quick stir and cover.
- Cook high pressure 25 minutes; natural release.
- Finally Remove bay leaf, garnish with parsley and serve over pasta, squasta or whatever you wish!

**Nutrition Facts Per Serving** Calories: 133 calories / Total Fat: 3g / Saturated Fat: 0.5g / Cholesterol: 57mg

## Instant Pot Shrimp Recipes
## Points Values: 5

### *Ingredients*

- ¼ cup butter & 1 cup rice
- 2Tbsp minced garlic & 1½ cups water or broth
- 1 can black beans, rinsed and drained & 1lb Frozen Shrimp (raw or cooked, just make sure it's frozen)
- 15-20 drops Young Living Lime Vitality Essential Oil , Fresh or freeze dried cilantro & salt and pepper to taste

### *Instructions*

- At first Set Instant Pot to "saute" and melt butter
- Next Add rice and cook until brown
- Then Add garlic, salt, and pepper and cook until fragrant
- After taht Add water and lime oil, then beans and shrimp
- Set Instant Pot to manual and cook for 5 minutes
- Finally Release the pressure manually and serve dish topped with cilantro

## Instant Pot Buffalo Chicken Dip

Prep Time 5 mins// Cook Time1 Hrs
Servings: 5 / Calories: 263kcal

### *Ingredients*

- 1lb chicken & ½ cup chicken broth
- 1 block cream cheese & 1 cup fat free sour cream
- 1 cup cooked shredded/diced chicken & ⅓ cup Frank's buffalo wing sauce
- 1 tsp taco seasoning , 1 tbsp water & ⅓ cup shredded cheddar cheese

### *Instructions*

- First To cook chicken, combine both ingredients in your Instant Pot, seal, cook for 15 minutes on high pressure. Do a quick release.
- Next Pour out onto a cutting board and shred or dice.
- Then Rinse/dry out your basin, then start steps to make buffalo dip.
- After that Let your cream cheese come to room temperature, then cube it.
- Combine cream cheese, sour cream, wing sauce, taco seasoning, chicken, and water in your Instant Pot.
- Seal the lid, and set for 5 minutes on high pressure.
- Vent, open the lid, and sprinkle in your cheese.
- Finally Stir thoroughly so that cheese is incorporated, then serve with chips, veggies, or pretzels.

**Nutrition Facts Per Serving** Calories: 263kcal / Carbohydrates: 3g Protein: 15g / Fat: 20g / Saturated Fat: 11g / Cholesterol: 83mg / Sodium: 994mg

# Buffalo Chicken Wings

Prep Time 5 mins// Cook Time 11 mins
Servings: 4 // **Points Values: 3**

## Ingredients

- 2 lbs . 2 large breasts partially defrosted chicken breast cut into strips (I've also used frozen chicken breasts, please see below) & 1/2 cup Franks Red Hot Sauce
- 1 tsp . cayenne pepper & 1 tsp . salt
- 2 tbsp . butter , 1 tsp . pepper & 1/4 cup Franks Red Hot Sauce for coating

## Instructions

- First Turn the Instant Pot to saute to melt the butter. When it is melted add in the chicken, salt, pepper, and cayenne pepper. Next Mix the chicken so that each piece is seasoned.
- I've also placed frozen chicken breasts in the Instant Pot, along with the other ingredients (minus butter), and cooked for 16 minutes. I cube the chicken after it's cooked and continue with the recipe.
- Then Add 1/2 cup hot sauce then stir the chicken so that it is coated.
- Lock the lid into place and turn the steam valve to sealing. Using the manual setting cook on high pressure for 8 minutes. If your chicken is fully defrosted cook for 7 minutes. I used partially defrosted chicken because it is easier to cut. Release the pressure using the quick release method.
- In a hurry? Drizzle warm sauce before serving and skip the last step!
- Finally Using tongs, remove the chicken from the Instant Pot and place on a baking sheet lined with aluminum foil.

Brush the chicken with the additional 1/4 cup hot sauce. Thicken the sauce by placing under the broiler for 3 minutes. Turn the chicken over and repeat on the other side. Let the chicken cool 5 minutes before serving. Goat cheese is tastes amazing spread on top.

**Nutrition Facts Per Serving** Weight Watchers, 1 Serving (Recipe Serves 4), 3 Freestyle Smart Points

# Instant Pot Chicken Tikka Masala with Cauliflower and Peas

Total Time: 25 minutes
Servings : 6, Serving Size: 3/4 cup // **Points Values: 5**

## Ingredients:

- 1 1/2 pounds skinless, boneless chicken thighs, cubed & 1 1/2 teaspoon kosher salt
- 1/2 tablespoon ghee, butter or coconut oil for df & 1/2 chopped onion
- 3 cloves garlic, minced & 1 teaspoon grated ginger root
- 1 teaspoon ground coriander & 1 teaspoon cumin
- 1/2 teaspoon turmeric & 1/2 teaspoon garam masala
- 1/4 teaspoon cayenne pepper & 1/4 teaspoon ground cardamom
- 14 ounce can diced tomatoes, drained & 2 cups cauliflower florets
- 1/2 cup frozen peas , 1/2 cup full fat canned coconut milk & 1/4 cup fresh cilantro leaves, for serving

## Instructions:

- First Season chicken with 1 teaspoon salt.
- Next Press saute button and melt the butter, add onion, garlic, ginger and 6 spices (from coriander to cardamom) and saute until the vegetables are soft and the spices are fragrant, about 2 to 3 minutes.
- Then Add the tomatoes and use an immersion to blend until smooth (or blend in the blender), add the chicken, remaining 1/2 teaspoon salt and stir, cook high pressure 15 minutes.

- Quick release, add the cauliflower and peas and cook 2 minutes on high pressure.
- Finally Quick release & stir in coconut milk and serve garnished with cilantro.

**Nutrition Facts Per Serving** Calories: 226 calories /Total Fat: 10g / Saturated Fat: g /Cholesterol: 3mg

## Macaroni and Cheese

Prep Time 5 mins // Cook Time 5 mins
Servings 8 // **Points Values : 8**

### *Ingredients*

- 12 ounces whole wheat shell pasta & 4 cups low-fat and low-sodium chicken stock
- 1 cup fat-free half and half & 6 slices Velveeta Original cheese slices
- 1/4 cup Parmesan grated & 1/4 cup Fat-Free Cheddar shredded
- 1 tablespoon margarine & 1 teaspoon garlic powder
- 1 teaspoon black pepper & 1 1/2 teaspoon salt

### *Instructions*

- First Pour pasta, half and half, and chicken stock into Instant Pot liner and stir.
- Next Place lid on Instant Pot and set to seal.
- Then Choose manual and set to 5 minutes.
- Allow to come to pressure, cook, and when complete NPR (natural pressure release) for 2 minutes. Release remaining pressure, and set to saute.
- Add in cheese slices, margarine, garlic powder, salt, and pepper and mix well. Stir consistently until completely melted.
- Finally Turn off saute feature and taste. May add salt and pepper to taste.

**Nutrition Facts Per Serving** Amount Per Serving (8 g) /Calories 243 Calories from Fat 45 /Total Fat 5g /Saturated Fat 1g /Cholesterol 8mg

# Buffalo Chicken Wings

Prep Time 5 mins // Cook Time 11 mins
Servings: 4 // **Points Values: 3**

## *Ingredients*

- 2 lbs. 2 large breasts partially defrosted chicken breast cut into strips (I've also used frozen chicken breasts, please see below) & 1/2 cup Franks Red Hot Sauce
- 1 tsp. cayenne pepper & 1 tsp. salt
- 2 tbsp. butter, 1 tsp. pepper & 1/4 cup Franks Red Hot Sauce for coating

## *Instructions*

- First Turn the Instant Pot to saute to melt the butter. When it is melted add in the chicken, salt, pepper, and cayenne pepper. Mix the chicken so that each piece is seasoned.
- Next I've also placed frozen chicken breasts in the Instant Pot, along with the other ingredients (minus butter), and cooked for 16 minutes. I cube the chicken after it's cooked and continue with the recipe.
- Then Add 1/2 cup hot sauce then stir the chicken so that it is coated.
- After that Lock the lid into place and turn the steam valve to sealing. Using the manual setting cook on high pressure for 8 minutes. If your chicken is fully defrosted cook for 7 minutes. I used partially defrosted chicken because it is easier to cut. Release the pressure using the quick release method.

- In a hurry? Drizzle warm sauce before serving and skip the last step!
- Finally Using tongs, remove the chicken from the Instant Pot and place on a baking sheet lined with aluminum foil. Brush the chicken with the additional 1/4 cup hot sauce. Thicken the sauce by placing under the broiler for 3 minutes. Turn the chicken over and repeat on the other side. Let the chicken cool 5 minutes before serving. Goat cheese is tastes amazing spread on top.

**Nutrition Facts Per Serving** Weight Watchers, 1 Serving (Recipe Serves 4), 3 Freestyle Smart Points

# Instant Pot Jambalaya

Prep Time 5 mins // Cook Time 20 mins
Servings: 4 // **Points Values: 7**

## *Ingredients*

- 225 g 1.5 cups andouille sausages, can be replaced with other smoky sausage or chorizo & 450 g 1 lb skinless chicken breast cut into bite sized pieces
- 2 tbsp oil & 1 onion peeled and chopped
- 2 peppers bell, deseeded and chopped & 2 stick celery sliced
- 1 tsp minced garlic & 1 ¾ cup chicken stock
- 1 tbsp soy sauce optional but oh so good (if gluten-free, use a gluten-free tamari soy sauce) & 400 g 14 oz tin chopped tomatoes
- 2 bay leaves & 1 tsp dried thyme & 1 tsp dried oregano
- 2 tsp Creole seasoning & 280 g 1.5 cups rice
- Salt & Cayenne pepper to taste
- 200 g 1.5 cups peeled deveined shrimps & To garnish
- Spring onions sliced & 2 tbsp chopped parsley

## *Instructions*

- At first In sauté mode, add half of the oil to the inner pot of the Instant Pot then add chicken breast. Sauté until browned, then remove and set aside.
- Next Add the sausage, cook, then remove and set aside.
- Then Add remaining oil and sauté the onions, peppers and celery until soft, then stir in garlic and switch off.
- After that Add the chicken stock and thoroughly deglaze the inner pot.
- In the next step Return the meats and the remainder of the ingredients through the cayenne pepper to the inner pot. Mix well.

- Close pot, set valve to sealing, select the manual or pressure cook button (dependent upon IP model), select high pressure and set the timer to 8 mins.
- When finished, do a QPR. Take insert out, add in shrimps and cover, letting residual heat cook for about 6-8 mins.
- Finally Serve garnished with parsley and spring onions.

## Recipe Notes

- Cook time does not include time to come up to pressure or for pressure to release.
- Andouille sausages are preferred, but go with any smoked sausage you have (eg polish smoked sausage or chorizo or even a mix).
- Make sure to deglaze well using the stock before cooking the rice.
- Do not use frozen shrimp. Use fresh, defrosted or already grilled (see the next tip) shrimps for this.
- We like actually adding already grilled shrimp to this. This makes it easier and quicker, just stir in the cooked shrimps and you are good to go.
- Reduce the Creole seasoning if you like less spice.
- I have also used 1 tbsp Cajun seasoning instead of Creole even though not authentic.

**Nutrition Facts Per Serving** Calories 388 Calories from Fat 126 / Total Fat 14g/ Saturated Fat 3g /Cholesterol 124mg / Sodium 795mg /Potassium 618mg

# Instant Pot BBQ Chicken Bowls

Prep Time 5 mins //Cook Time 20 mins
Servings: 4 // **Points Values:3**

## Ingredients

- 2 boneless skinless chicken breasts & ½ cup sugar free BBQ Sauce
- ½ cup water & 1 tbsp dehydrated onion flake
- 1 clove minced garlic & 1 box zucchini spirals
- 15 oz can black beans & 1 cup frozen corn thawed
- 2 oz pepper jack cheese & 2 scallions

## Instructions

- First Place the chicken breasts in the Instant Pot liner.
- Next Mix the bbq sauce, water, onion flakes and minced garlic in a bowl and pour over the chicken.
- Then Lock lid, set vent to sealing, and press manual high pressure for 8 minutes.
- After that Cook zucchini spirals in a skillet with salt and pepper for about 7-8 minutes.
- In the next step When Instant Pot beeps, let the pressure release naturally for 10 minutes.
- Remove chicken, and slice.
- Place zucchini spirals, black beans, corn, and chicken on a plate or in a bowl.
- Finally Sprinkle with pepper jack cheese and scallions.

**Nutrition Facts Per Serving** 3 Freestyle SmartPoints per bowl.

# Spanish Rice with Chicken

Prep Time 20 mins // Cook Time 9 mins
Servings : 4 // **Points Values: 1**

## *Ingredients*

- 1 tbsp. olive oil & 1/2 an onion chopped
- 1 large jalapeño chopped & 1 tbsp. minced garlic
- 1/2 tsp cumin & 1/2 tsp chili powder
- 1/2 tsp paprika & 1/2 tsp salt
- 2 tbsp. chopped cilantro & 4 boneless chicken thighs
- 4 cups cauliflower florets , 2 tbsp. tomato paste & 1/2 cup chicken broth

## *Instructions*

- First Turn the Instant Pot to sauté and add the olive oil. When the oil is hot sauté the onions, jalapeños, garlic, and cilantro for about 1 minutes. Add the cumin, chili powder, paprika, and salt and mix around.
- Next add in the chicken and chicken broth. Lock the lid into place and turn the pressure valve to sealing. Cook on high pressure using manual for 9 minutes. Release pressure using the quick release method.
- Then Remove the lid and place a steaming basket over the chicken. Add the cauliflower florets to the steaming basket. Lock the lid into place and cook on high pressure again for 1 minute. Release the pressure using the quick release method.
- Carefully remove the steaming basket full of cauliflower. Using a fork or tongs remove the chicken and set aside. There will be about 1/4 cup liquid at the bottom of the Instant Pot. Strain the liquid from the onions and jalapenos, leaving about 2 tbsp. of liquid and the onions and jalapeños in the Instant Pot.

- Add the cauliflower back into the Instant Pot. Use a mash potato masher to break the cauliflower into rice like chunks. Stir in the tomato paste to give the cauliflower rice a nice orange color.
- Finally Serve the rice immediately and top it with the chicken, fresh tomatoes, limes, and more cilantro.

# Spicy Beef and Broccoli Stir Fry

Prep Time 20 mins// Cook Time 20 mins
Servings: 4 // **Points Values: 4**

## *Ingredients*

- 3 Tbsp dry sherry & 3 Tbsp low sodium soy sauce
- 4 large garlic cloves minced & 1 tsp Asian sesame oil dark
- ¼ tsp red pepper flakes & ½ pound flank or skirt steak trimmed and cut into strips
- 1 tsp cornstarch & 1 Tbsp canola oil
- 4 cups broccoli florets & 1/4 cup of beef broth.

## *Instructions*

- At first Stir together sherry, soy sauce, garlic, sesame oil, red pepper flakes in 1 cup glass measuring cup.
- Next Transfer 1/2 of mixture to a large Ziploc bag and add beef. Seal bag and turn to coat beef. Refrigerate up to 2 hours to marinate.
- Then Add cornstarch and equal parts cold water to make a slurry. Stir until smooth. Depending on how much thickening your sauce needs...you can make a larger amount of slurry by combining equal amounts of cornstarch and cold water.
- After that Put 1 tablespoon of Oil in the instant pot on saute mode.
- In the next step Dump the marinated beef and sauce from the ziploc bag into the pot and sear it, till it no longer pink.
- Add rest of the sauce and beef broth and pressure cook on HIGH for 5 minutes.
- Once the IP beeps, release the steam using the "quick release" process.
- Turn it back on the saute mode and add the broccoli.

- Let it simmer in the sauce for 5 minutes till the broccoli is cooked, but still crunchy.
- Add the cornstarch slurry and let til simmer for another minute, till the sauce becomes thick and it coats the meat and the veggies.
- Finally Server hot with Brown rice or with Weight Watchers Cauliflower Fried Rice.

***Recipe Notes :*** 4 freestyle smartpoints per serving. Makes approximately 4 cups so serving size is one cup

**Nutrition Facts Per Serving** Calories 343 Calories from Fat 81 / Total Fat 9g 14% / Total Carbohydrates 47g 16% / Dietary Fiber 1g 4% / Sugars 33g

## Instant Pot Beef Stew

Prep Time 15 mins// Cook Time 40 mins
Servings: 8 // **Points Values: 3**

### Ingredients

- 1 lb lean beef cubes & Salt and pepper to taste
- 1 teaspoon Olive oil ,3 cups beef broth & ½ teaspoon of dried oregano ,1 bay leaf
- 2 cloves garlic minced , 1 15 ounce can tomato sauce
- 1 cup carrots chopped & 1 medium onion chopped
- 1 cup of celery chopped & 1 cup of corn frozen, fresh or canned--drained
- 1.5 cups red potatoes cubed with skins on or off

### Instructions

- At first Click Sauté on the Instant Pot and add Olive oil, garlic, onions, dried oregano, and meat and brown meat for about 4 minutes.
- Next Follow by the carrots, celery, salt and pepper and sauté for another 4 to 5 minutes.
- Then Turn off Sauté and add the rest of the ingredients into the Instant Pot.
- Finally Hit the Manual button and 17 minutes and let it release naturally. My pot took about 25-30 minutes to do this process. I prefer my meat to be really tender. You can add more time if desired to make sure the meat is nice and tender!

**Recipe Notes :** You can make this in a slow cooker too. Just add all the ingredients and cook on low for 8 hours or until meat is really tender.

**Nutrition Facts Per Serving** This recipe serves around 8 and is 3 Freestyle SmartPoints per cup serving.

# Homemade Baked Beans Recipe

Prep time: 5 mins // Cook time: 1 hour
Serves: 10 // **Points Values:3**

## Ingredients

- 1 cup dry pinto beans & ½ cup dry black beans
- ½ cup dry dark red kidney beans & 6 cups vegetable broth
- 3 cups water, onion, diced & 1 teaspoon garlic powder, 1 teaspoon onion powder
- 2 cups green enchilada sauce (no sugar added and fat-free) & ¼ cup brown mole sauce, ¾ cups barbecue sauce

## Instructions

- At first Combine all ingredients in your Instant Pot Liner and stir to combine.
- Next Place lid and set to seal.
- Then Set to high pressure and cook for 60 minutes.
- Once cooking cycle has completed, allow the Instant Pot to naturally pressure release.
- Finally Remove lid and stir to combine. Taste for flavor. You may wish to add salt or pepper for more flavor.

**Nutrition Facts Per Serving** Makes 10 servings (1 1/2 cups per serving) 3 SmartPoints on FreeStyle, Flex, and Your Way Plans 7 SmartPoints on Beyond the Scale

# Mexican Spiced Instant Pot Cauliflower Soup

Prep Time 5 mins// Cook Time 7 mins // **Points Values:0**

## *Ingredients*

- 1 tbsp olive oil & 2 onion peeled and finely chopped & 1 pepper, deseeded and finely chopped
- 1 bay leaf optional & 1 tsp garlic puree
- 1.5 tsp smoked paprika & 1.5 tsp ground cumin
- Chilli to taste & 1 head of a large cauliflower approx 675 g /1.5lb cut into florets
- 750 ml 3 cups vegetable stock & Salt

## *Instructions*

- At first Switch the Instant Pot on to the saute setting and add the oil to the Instant Pot Insert and saute the onions, peppers and bay leaf if using for 4-5 mins until the onion is soft.
- Next Switch off the heat and stir in the garlic, paprika, cumin and chilli.
- Then Mix in the cauliflower florets, vegetable stock and salt.
- Cover your Instant Pot, set the vent to 'sealing,' select the manual or pressure cook button (dependent upon IP model), select high pressure and set the timer to 7 mins.
- When done allow the pot to NPR for 15 mins before releasing the rest of the steam using quick release.
- Let cool for a few mins, before removing bay leaf and pureeing with an immersion blender.
- Finally Garnish and serve.

**Nutrition Facts Per Serving** Calories 120 Calories from Fat 36 / Total Fat 4g / Sodium 806mg / Potassium 682mg / Total Carbohydrates 18mg / Dietary Fiber 5g / Sugars 8g

# Instant Pot Spicy Tomato Sauce

Prep Time 5 mins // Cook Time 15 mins
Servings: 4 // **Points Values:1**

## Ingredients

- 1 Tbsp extra-virgin olive oil & 3 large garlic cloves minced
- ¼-1/2 tsp red pepper flakes
- 28 ounce can whole tomatoes in juice drained and broken up (fire-roasted tomatoes are even better!) , ½ tsp salt & ¼ tsp pepper

## Instructions

- At first Place all the ingredients into the Instant Pot.
- Next Pressure cook for the ingredients for 15 minutes and then let it release naturally.
- Then Using a hand blender puree the sauce until it is a consistency you like! I don't like mine to be chunky...so I blend until smooth.

## Recipe Notes

- Use canned fire roasted tomatoes for even more flavor!
- You can use less or no red pepper flakes to reduce the heat!
- Store in refrigerator in a jar with lid...double the batch to have extra sauce!
- Be sure to remember that total cook time will vary based on how long it takes to release the pressure!
- If you are doing Weight Watchers this recipe is 1 Freestyle SmartPoint per cup serving!

**Nutrition Facts Per Serving** Calories: 102 cal

## Instant Pot Honey Garlic Chicken

Prep Time: 5 Min // Cook Time: 25 Min
Serving Size: 6 // **Points Values:6**

### *Ingredients*

- 2 lbs. boneless skinless chicken thighs & 1/3 cup low sodium soy sauce
- 1/4 cup ketchup (no sugar added) & 3 tbsp. Honey, 4 garlic cloves, minced

### *Instructions*

- At first Add the chicken thighs to the bottom of the slow cooker. Mix together the remaining ingredients to create the sauce.
- Next Pour over the chicken and stir. Cook on manual mode for 20 minutes. Once it is finished cooking, use the quick release.
- Then Shred the chicken using two forks. If needed, you can thicken up the sauce using a touch of cornstarch, although normally I don't need it. It will depend on the liquid content of your chicken thighs,

**Nutrition Facts Per Serving** Calories 234 / Calories from Fat 1 /Protein 30g

# Instant Pot Jerk Chicken Soup

Prep Time 20 mins // Cook Time 15 mins
Servings: 6// **Points Values:0**

## *Ingredients*

- ¼ tsp ground all spice & ¼ tsp ground cayenne pepper
- ½ tsp ground ginger & ½ tsp black pepper
- 1 lbs. skinless chicken breast cut into one-inch cubes & 1 clove garlic minced
- 1 medium onion chopped & 1 can of can diced tomatoes with green chilies drained
- 1 can of black beans drained and rinsed , 5 cups of fat-free chicken broth & ½ tbsp. of salt & Fresh lime--squeezed or 2 tbsp. of cilantro

## *Instructions*

- First take your pressure cooker pot and combine the all spice, cayenne pepper, ginger, garlic salt, and pepper and mix the spices together.
- Next add the chicken breast cubes to the spice bowl and coat the chicken in the spices.
- Let the chicken sit in the bowl for around 15 minutes so it gets nice and marinated.
- Go ahead and add the garlic, onion, tomatoes, black beans and chicken broth to the pot with the coated chicken cubes.
- Stir everything together.
- Last just set your Instant Pot to manual and set it for 15 minutes.

**Nutrition Facts Per Serving** : Serving size is 6 cups. The whole pot of soup is 1

# Protein Packed Chicken Stew

Prep Time: 10 mins// Cook Time: 20 mins
Servings: 6 cups // **Points Values:1**

## *Ingredients*

- 1 Tablespoon olive oil & 1 medium onion chopped
- 2 Tablespoons garlic minced & 3 stalks celery chopped
- 3 small carrots chopped & 1 pound small red potatoes corsely chopped
- 15oz can diced tomatoes with juices & 15oz can red kidney beans drained and rinsed
- 1 cup low-sodium chicken broth & 1 pound boneless chicken breasts
- 1 teaspoon dried oregano 7 1 Tablespoon balsamic vinegar
- 1 teaspoon red pepper flakes , 1 teaspoon salt & 1/2 teaspoon black pepper

## *Instructions*

- At first Heat the olive oil on SAUTE mode of your electric pressure cooker with the lid off. Next Add the onion, garlic, celery and carrots and stir. Then Cook the veggies for about 5 minutes, or until the onion is translucent and the garlic is fragrant.
- After that Add the potatoes, diced tomatoes, beans, broth. Lay the chicken on top of the veggies and add the oregano and red pepper flakes over the chicken. Season everything with salt and pepper.
- Finally Secure the lid and select MANUAL mode. Cook at high pressure for 10 minutes. Use a natural release when the cooking is complete (this takes 10 - 15 minutes). Remove the chicken breast and shred. Add the balsamic vinegar and stir everything together. Return the chicken to the stew, stir and serve immediately.

***Notes*** **:** You can use the Quick Release option on your electric pressure cooker, if you are pressed for time. You can also use the SOUP setting, if applicable, for this recipe. Set the timer to 10 minutes using this setting and proceed with the recipe.

**Nutrition Facts Per Serving** Calories: 307kcal //Carbohydrates: 32g / Protein: 23.1g //Fat: 10.2g / Saturated Fat: 2.6g // Cholesterol: 48.4mg

# Split Pea Soup with Ham

Total Time: 25 minutes
Servings : 8, Serving Size: 1 cup // **Points Values:1**

## Ingredients:

- 1 lb dry green split peas, 1 tsp olive oil & 2 large carrots, peeled and diced
- 1 medium onion, diced, 1/4 cup diced celery & 2 cloves garlic, minced, leftover ham bone
- 1 tbsp Better Than Bouillon or 1 cube* , 1 bay leaf, 6 cups water & 4 ounces leftover ham, diced, chopped chives for garnish

## Instructions:

- At first Rinse peas under cold water.
- Next In a pressure cooker, add oil, onions, carrots, celery and garlic and saute 4-5 minutes. Add ham bone, peas, water, chicken bouillon and bay leaf. Cover and cook high pressure for 15 minutes. Let the pressure release naturally then open, remove the bone and bay leaf and stir, the soup will thicken as it stands.
- Then Saute the ham on a hot skillet if desired and use for garnish on the soup with chives.
- Finally To make without a pressure cooker, add 2 more cups water and simmer covered on low for 2 hours.

**Nutrition Facts Per Serving** Calories: 182 calories // Total Fat: 1.5g / Saturated Fat: g / Cholesterol: 0mg

## Spaghetti Squash Pad Thai (Low Carb)

Prep Time: 10 mins// Cook Time: 35 mins
Servings: 4 // **Points Values:13**

### Ingredients

- 1 medium onion sliced ,2 eggs & 2 carrots grated,1 tbsp olive oil
- 1.5 - 2 lbs. thinly cut chicken breasts frozen & Cilantro, lime wedges , toasted peanuts

Sauce: 2 tbsp fish sauce, 1 tbsp rice vinegar, 2 cloves garlic, 3 tbsp honey

### Instructions

- At first Add 2 cups water and a trivet to the Instant Pot insert.
- Next Using a knife cut a dozen venting slits into the spaghetti squash. Then Place the spaghetti squash on the trivet and arrange the chicken around the spaghetti squash.
- After that Close the lid and turn the pressure valve to sealing. Cook on high pressure using manual for 15 minutes. Let the pressure release naturally.
- In the next step Remove the spaghetti squash and chicken from the Instant Pot using a trivet. Place the spaghetti squash on a large plate or cutting board and cut it in half while it is still hot. I was able to slice my knife right through the squash. Chop the chicken into bite sized cubes.
- While the spaghetti squash is cooling rinse out the Instant Pot liner and turn the Instant Pot back on to sauté. Add the oil and sauté the onions and carrots for 2-3 minutes. Push the onions and carrots to the side and crack the eggs on the empty side of the Instant Pot. Scramble the eggs and then mix them together with the onions and carrots. Turn the Instant Pot to keep warm then add the chicken back into the Instant Pot.
- Mix together the sauce ingredients in a small bowl until the honey is dissolved then pour it over the chicken and onions in the Instant Pot. Give it a good stir and then let it sit while you shred the spaghetti squash to absorb some of the flavor.

- Finally Add the spaghetti squash noodles to the Instant Pot and mix it up. Serve while still warm topped with cilantro, lime, and crushed peanuts.

**Recipe Notes :** My store only had huge spagetti sqaush, but it fit in the Instant Pot after I trimmed the edges some.

**Nutrition Facts Per Serving** Servings Per Recipe: 3 / Serving Size: 1 serving / Calories 376.8 / Total Fat 12.7 g / Saturated Fat 2.7 g

## Chickpea Sweet Potato Stew

Prep Time:15 minutes // Cook Time:4 hours
Servings : 6, Serving Size: 1 1/2 cups // **Points Values:3**

### Ingredients:

- 1 medium yellow onion, chopped & 2 15 oz cans garbanzo beans, drained
- 1 pound sweet potatoes, peeled and chopped & 1 tablespoon garlic, minced
- 1/2 teaspoon Kosher salt & 1/4 teaspoon coarse ground black pepper
- 1 teaspoon ground ginger & 1 1/2 teaspoons ground cumin
- 1 teaspoon ground coriander & 1/4 teaspoon ground cinnamon
- 4 cups vegetable broth, fat free & 4 cups fresh baby spinach

### Instructions:

- At first Add the ingredients together except for the spinach and cook on high pressure for 8 minutes.
- Next Quick release, stir in the spinach and let it sit 2 minutes covered, until wilted.
- Finally (You can also sweat the garlic and onions first, but if doing so add a teaspoon of olive oil. This will give you the best results)

**Nutrition Facts Per Serving** Calories: 165 calories / Total Fat: 2.2g /Saturated Fat: 1.4g /Cholesterol: 0mg

## Barbacoa Beef (Instant Pot)

Total Time: 1 hour 20 minutes
Servings : 9, Size: 4 oz  //  **Points Values:3**

### Ingredients:

- 5 cloves garlic,1/2 medium onion & 1 lime, juice, 2-4 tbsp chiptoles in adobo sauce & (to taste),1 tbsp ground cumin & 1 tbsp ground oregano
- 1/2 tsp ground cloves, 1 cup water & 3 lbs beef eye of round or bottom round roast, all fat trimmed
- 2 1/2 teaspoons kosher salt ,black pepper & 1 tsp oil , 3 bay leaves

### Instructions:

- At first Place garlic, onion, lime juice, cumin, oregano, chipotles, cloves and water in a blender and puree until smooth.
- Next Trim all the fat off meat, cut into 3-inch pieces. Season with 2 teaspoons salt and black pepper. Then Heat the pressure cooker on high (use saute button for Instant Pot), when hot add the oil and brown the meat, in batches on all side, about 5 minutes. Add the sauce from the blender and bay leaves, cover and cook on high pressure until the meat is tender and easily shreds with 2 forks, about 1 hour. (in my Instant Pot I cooked it 65 minutes). (If you're making this on the stove, simmer it on low at least 4 hours, adding more water as needed to make sure it doesn't dry out.)
- Finally Once cooked and the meat is tender, remove the meat and place in a dish. Shred with two forks, and reserve the liquid for later (discard the bay leaf). Return the shredded meat to the pot, add 1/2 teaspoon salt or to taste, 1/2 tsp cumin and 1 1/2 cups of the reserved liquid.

**Nutrition Facts Per Serving** Calories: 153 calories //Total Fat: 4.5g
Saturated Fat: g //Cholesterol: 44mg

# Turkey Meatball Stroganoff

Total Time:40 mins //Prep Time:10 mins
Servings : 4, Size: 5 meatballs // **Points Values:7**

## Ingredients:

- 1 teaspoon olive oil, divided & 1/2 cup chopped onion
- 1 pound 93% ground turkey & 1/3 cup whole wheat seasoned breadcrumbs
- 1 large egg, beaten & 1/4 cup chopped parsley, divided
- 3 tbsp fat free milk & 3/4 tsp kosher salt
- black pepper, to taste & 3/4 cups water
- 1/2 cup light sour cream & 2 tbsp all purpose flour
- 2 teaspoons tomato paste & 2 teaspoons beef Bouillon (I like Better Than Bouillon)
- 1/2 teaspoon Worcestershire sauce & 1/2 teaspoon paprika
- 8 ounces sliced Cremini mushrooms & 1 sprig fresh thyme

## *Instructions*

- First Heat a large nonstick skillet or set the Instant Pot to saute and spray with oil; saute the onions over medium heat until golden, stirring 2 to 3 minutes. Remove and divide in two.
- Next In a large bowl, combine half of the sautéed onions with the ground turkey, bread crumbs, egg, 2 tbsp of the parsley, milk, 3/4 tsp salt and black pepper. Gently shape into 20 meatballs.
- Then In a blender combine the water, sour cream, flour, tomato paste, boullion, Worcestershire sauce and paprika, blend until smooth.

- After that Heat the skillet or Instant Pot back on saute, add the oil and brown half of the meatballs without disturbing (in two batches) about 2 minutes until no longer sticks, turn and brown an additional 2 minutes, set aside on a dish and repeat with remaining meatballs.
- In the next step Place all the meatballs and remaining onion into the Instant pot, Slow Cooker or a large saucepan and pour the sauce over the meatballs along with the thyme and mushrooms.
- Finally Cook on high pressure 10 minutes. Let the pressure release on it's own. When done, discard thyme, add the chopped parsley and serve over your favorite noodles.

**Nutrition Facts Per Serving** Amount Per Serving:Freestyle Points: 7Points +: 8 Calories: 310 calories

# WW INSTANT POT DINNER RECIPES

## Garlicky Cuban Pork

Total Time: 80 minutes plus marinade time
Servings : 10, Serving Size: a little over 3 oz // **Points Values:5**

### *Ingredients:*
- 3 lb boneless pork shoulder blade roast, lean, all fat removed & 6 cloves garlic
- juice of 1 grapefruit (about 2/3 cup) & juice of 1 lime
- 1/2 tablespoon fresh oregano & 1/2 tablespoon cumin
- 1 tablespoon kosher salt & 1 bay leaf
- lime wedges, for serving & chopped cilantro, for serving
- hot sauce, for serving , tortillas, optional for serving & salsa, optional for serving

### *Instructions:*
- PRESSURE COOKER: First Cut the pork in 4 pieces and place in a bowl.
- Next In a small blender or mini food processor, combine garlic, grapefruit juice, lime juice, oregano, cumin and salt and blend until smooth.
- Then Pour the marinade over the pork and let it sit room temperature 1 hour or refrigerated as long as overnight.
- After that Transfer to the pressure cooker, add the bay leaf, cover and cook high pressure 80 minutes. Let the pressure release naturally.
- Remove pork and shred using two forks.
- Finally Remove liquid from pressure cooker, reserving then place the pork back into pressure cooker. Add about 1 cup of the liquid (jus) back, adjust the salt as needed and keep warm until you're ready to eat.

**Nutrition Facts Per Serving** Calories: 213 calories / Total Fat: 9.5g / Saturated Fat: 0g / Cholesterol: 91mg

# Healthy Tuscan Chicken Pasta

Prep Time 10 mins // Cook Time 4 mins
Servings: 6 // **Points Values:7**

## Ingredients

- 3 cups chicken broth , 1/2 cup sun-dried tomatoes (no oil) & 1/2 tbsp Italian seasoning
- 1 tbsp minced garlic & 2 lbs. chicken breast diced into 1-inch cubes
- 12 oz whole wheat noodles (I used one 12 oz. box) & 2 cups baby spinach
- 3/4 cup Fat Free Greek Yogurt & 3/4 cup Fat Free cottage cheese
- 2/3 cup parmesan , 1/4 cup fresh basil 1 tsp dried & 1/2 tsp salt , 1/4 tsp pepper

## Instructions

- At first Turn the Instant Pot to sauté mode. Add the sun-dried tomatoes, garlic, Italian seasoning, salt, and pepper. Sauté for 30 seconds until fragrant.
- Next add the chicken to the Instant Pot. Brown the chicken for 1-2 minutes, this will keep the chicken from sticking together while cooking.
- Then Add the pasta and chicken broth to the Instant Pot, if needed stir the pasta to make sure all the pasta is covered by the liquid.
- Close the lid and turn the pressure valve to sealing. Cook on high pressure using the manual setting for 4 minutes. Let the pressure naturally release.
- While the pasta is cooking blend together the cottage cheese and Greek yogurt to make a cream sauce. Set it aside until ready to use.

- Remove the Instant Pot lid and stir the noodles and pasta. While the pasta is still hot add the parmesan cheese, spinach, and basil. Mix the pasta until the cheese melts and the spinach wilts.
- Finally Pour the blended cream sauce over the pasta. Stir it until all the pasta is covered in sauce. Serve immediately.

**Nutrition Facts Per Serving** Calories: 364kcal //Carbohydrates: 39g /Protein: 39g / Fat: 6g //Saturated Fat: 2g //Cholesterol: 80mg

## Shredded Mexican Chicken

Prep Time 5 mins // Cook Time 15 mins
Servings: 6 // **Points Values: 4**

### Ingredients

- 2 lbs boneless, skinless chicken breasts, frozen & 1.2 c non-fat, low-sodium chicken broth
- 2 10-oz cans Rotel fire-roasted diced tomatoes and green chiles, undrained & 2 15-oz cans black beans, rinsed and drained
- 3-4 garlic cloves, minced & 1 small jalapeno pepper, finely diced
- 1 T hickory-flavored liquid smoke (if you leave this out, you'll be fine) & 2 tsp ground cumin
- 1 T chili powder & 1 tsp smoked paprika
- 2 tsp dried oregano & 1 tsp cayenne pepper (leave this out if it's too spicy)
- salt and pepper, to taste , 2 limes, quartered
- 1.4 c fresh cilantro, chopped & Place the frozen chicken in your Instant Pot. Add all ingredients to the pot.

### Instructions

- First Lock the lid into place and make sure the pressure valve is set to seal. Set on manual for 16 minutes at high pressure. Next Let the pressure release naturally.
- Then Drain any liquid and shred the chicken.
- Finally Serve with letuce wraps, plain, over rice or on corn tortillas.

**Nutrition Facts Per Serving** Calories 218 Calories from Fat 36 / Total Fat 4g / Saturated Fat 1g / Cholesterol 108mg / Sodium 437mg

# BBQ Pulled Pork Recipe

Cook Time 15 mins Servings: 4 // **Points Values:7**

## Ingredients

- 1 pound of uncooked lean pork tenderloin sliced & 1/2 cup Sugar Free BBQ sauce of choice
- 2 cups packaged coleslaw mix & 2 Tbsp light mayo
- 1 tsp apple cider vinegar , 1/4 tsp stevia or less just for sweetness and taste & 4 whole wheat bread thins

## Instructions

- At first Cut and cube the pork tenderloin, then place in the crock pot on low for about 4 hours. Then remain on warm until you are ready to eat your meal. The internal temp needed for pork is 145 degrees Fahrenheit.
- Next Add BBQ sauce to meat in crock pot when you start cooking.
- After that Mix coleslaw with mayo, apple cider vinegar and stevia in a bowl. Set aside.
- In the next step Once meat is cooked and before serving, simply shred meat in the crock pot with a fork.
- Finally Place 3 oz of BBQ pulled pork with 1/3 cup of slaw mix on your whole wheat bread thins and you are good to go!

**Nutrition Facts Per Serving** Calories 286 Calories from Fat 45 / Total Fat 5g 8% // Saturated Fat 1g 5% // Cholesterol 74mg 25% //Sodium 606mg 25% //Potassium 788mg 23% //Sugars 13g //Protein 29g

# Instant Pot Goulash

Prep Time 5 mins // Cook Time 10 mins
Servings: 8 // **Points Values:3**

## *Ingredients*
- 1 lb ground turkey & 1 tbsp. minced garlic
- 2 1/2 tbsp Italian seasoning & 1 tbsp. minced onions
- 1 tsp. salt & 2 bay leaves
- 1 chopped zucchini & 1 cup chopped red and green bell peppers
- 8 oz. whole wheat pasta, 1 - 14 oz can crushed tomatoes OR jarred sauce & 1 can water (you'll be filling the tomato can with water)

## *Instructions*
- At first Turn Instant Pot to saute and brown the ground turkey.
- Next Add your 1 tbsp. garlic, 1 tbsp. minced onions, 2 1/2 tbsp. Italian seasoning, 1 tsp. salt, and 2 bay leaves. Toss in your 1 chopped zucchini and 1 cup of red and green bell peppers.
- Then Mix so that the seasonings and veggies are distributed.
- After that Pour the 8 ounces of dry whole wheat pasta, can of crushed tomatoes (or a jar of pasta sauce), and fill the can back up with water and pour that over the vegetables.
- In the next step Stir until the pasta is fully mixed with the sauce. Lock the lid into place and turn the pressure valve to sealing. Cook on high pressure using the manual function for 10 minutes. Use the quick release method to release the pressure. Give it a stir and let the goulash cool for a few minutes–it's super hot!
- Finally Top with cheese if desired and serve.

**Nutrition Facts Per Serving** Calories: 501kcal, Carbohydrates: 52.2g, Protein: 40.4g, Fat: 16.7g.

# Roasted Chicken Breast & Vegetables

Prep time: 10 mins // Cook time: 40 mins
Serves: 4 // **Points Values:7**

## *Ingredients*

- ½ Chicken or 2 Bone-In Chicken Breasts & 2 Cups Carrots
- 8 medium new potatoes (red or yellow) & 1 cup pearl onions (or 1 onion chopped)
- ½ Cup Chicken Broth & 1 Spring Rosemary
- 1 Spring Thyme , 2 cloves garlic, minced & 1 teaspoon salt , 1 teaspoon black pepper

## *Instructions*

- At first Season chicken breasts with salt and pepper
- Next Spread olive oil over bottom of Instant Pot and pour chicken broth into bottom of Instant Pot
- Then Place chicken on top of the broth and cover with onions, thyme, rosemary, and garlic.
- After that Top with carrots and potatoes (you may wish to season with salt and pepper)
- In the next step Place Instant Pot lid on and set to seal.
- Meanwhile Set to the Meat Setting for 20 minutes.
- In the meantime Allow to NPR. Remove from Instant Pot.
- Finally For those who want crispy skin, remove the chicken from the Instant Pot and place under the broiler for 5 minutes.

**Nutrition Facts Per Serving** Serving Size: 4 ounces chicken (skin removed), 1/2 cup potatoes, 1/2 cup carrots / SmartPoints: 7 Per Serving

## Instant Pot Vegetable Noodle Soup

Prep 10 mins// Cook 11 mins
Servings: 4 // **Points Values:4**

### *Ingredients*

- 1 onion, finely chopped & 1 large carrot, diced
- 1/2 a small sweet potato - diced & 1 clove of garlic, crushed
- 1/2 cup of frozen sweetcorn & 1 tbs of tomato paste
- 1 tsp of paprika & 1/4 tsp of garlic powder
- 1/4 tsp of chilli powder & pinch of dried basil, oregano, thyme and parsley
- salt and black pepper & 5 cups (1.2 litres) of vegetable or chicken stock
- 100g (3.5oz) of uncooked pasta of choice & 4 handfuls of spinach , spray oil

### *Instructions*

- At first Set instant pot to saute mode
- Next Once hot, spray with spray oil, add onion, garlic and carrots and fry for 2 minutes to soften.
- Then Mix in the sweet potato, tomato paste and spices and herbs and stir to coat.
- After that Add the stock, sweetcorn and pasta, add lid, close valve and set to 8 mins high pressure.
- In the next step Once cooking is complete, do a quick pressure release and stir through the spinach. Season as needed with salt and black pepper.
- Optional: Finally top with a little grated parmesan as part of your Healthy Extra A allowance.

**Nutrition Facts Per Serving** Amount Per Serving, Calories 171

# Vegan Instant Pot Mushroom Soup

Prep Time 15 mins// Cook Time 25 mins
Serves : 4 // **Points Values:3**

## Ingredients

- 2 tsp olive oil & 1 medium onion, chopped
- 1 large celery stalk, chopped & 1 large carrot, peeled & chopped
- 4 garlic cloves, minced & 8 oz. crimini mushrooms, sliced
- 8 oz. shiitake mushrooms, stems removed, sliced & 1 tsp dried thyme
- 1/2 tsp ground pepper & 3 cups high-quality vegetable broth
- 1/2 tsp kosher salt & 2/3 cup lite coconut milk

## Instructions

- At first Set the Instant Pot to Saute mode. Heat the olive oil, then add the onion, celery and carrots. Saute the vegetables, stirring occasionally, until starting to soften, 3 to 4 minutes.
- Next Add the garlic, crimini and shiitake mushrooms, thyme and pepper. Cook until the mushrooms are starting to release their liquid, 2 to 3 minutes. Stir in the broth and salt.
- Then Put the lid on the Instant Pot, close the steam vent and set to HIGH pressure using the manual setting. Decrease the time to 10 minutes. It will take the Instant Pot about 10 minutes to reach pressure.
- In the next step Once the time is expired, carefully release the steam using the quick release valve.
- Meanwhile Transfer half of the soup to the blender, add the coconut milk, hold on the top and blend until almost smooth (leave a little bit of texture), stopping the blender and opening the lid occasionally to release the steam. Transfer the pureed soup to a pot or bowl. Repeat with the second half of the soup.
- Finally If the soup needs to be reheated, return it to the Instant Pot and heat gently over the Saute mode. Serve.

**Nutrition Facts Per Serving** Serving Size 1 1/2 cups // Amount Per Serving As Served / Calories 108.3cal // Calories from fat 45

# HEALTHY BANANA CAKE RECIPE

Prep time: 15 mins // Cook time: 35 mins
Serves: 16 // **Points Values:6**

## Ingredients

- cup shortening (you can replace with butter or margarine, but points change) & 1 cup Swerve granulated sweetener
- 2 eggs
- 1 cup mashed ripe bananas, usually 2-3 bananas & 1 teaspoon vanilla extract
- 1½ cups all-purpose flour & 1 teaspoon baking soda
- ¼ cup low-fat buttermilk & Ingredients for Cream Cheese Frosting
- 2 SmartPoints per serving when divided by 16 & 4 ounces light cream cheese, softened
- ¼ cup butter, softened , 2 teaspoons vanilla extract & 1 cup Swerve confectioners sweetener

## Instructions

- At first Preheat oven to 325 degrees (dark pan) or 350 degrees (glass pan).
- Next Spray cake pan/casserole with nonstick cooking spray and set aside
- Then With a mixer, cream shortening and Swerve sweetener together until fluffy (approximately 3 minutes).
- After that Add eggs, bananas, and vanilla extract to the mixture and beat well.
- In the next step In a small bowl, combine the all-purpose flour and baking soda mixing well.
- Meanwhile Add flour and buttermilk to the liquid mixture and beat until just combined.
- Pour into a prepared cake pan.
- Bake for 20-35 minutes depending on pan choice (dark pan for 25-35 minutes, glass pan for 20-30 minutes). Check with a toothpick in the center to see if done completely.

- Remove from the oven and allow to cool completely.
- If adding cream cheese frosting, follow directions below:
- Add cream cheese, butter, and vanilla to a mixer and beat well until smooth. Slowly mix in the Swerve confectioners sugar until combined. Increase the speed and whip until you have a frosting consistency you prefer. Usually 2-3 minutes. You may add a bit of water or more confectioners sugar as needed to get the texture you prefer.
- Finally Place icing in a piping bag and pipe in small amounts onto each square of the cake prior to serving.

**Nutrition Facts Per Serving** Calories: 199 kcal, Carbohydrates: 22 g, Protein: 2.8 g

## Healthy Beef Stew

Prep Time: 15 Min // Cook Time: 40 Min
Serving Size: 1.5 cups // **Points Values:8**

### Ingredients

- 1 1/2 lb lean stewing beef, cut into 1-inch chunks & 2 tbsp flour
- 1 tbsp vegetable oil & 3 cups beef broth
- 2 tbsp Worcestershire sauce & 3 garlic cloves, minced
- 2 bay leaves, 1 tsp salt & 1 tsp sugar, 1 tsp paprika
- 1/2 tsp pepper, 1/2 tsp thyme, 1 lb carrots, chopped, 1 lb potatoes, chopped & 1 onion, diced, 2 celery ribs, chopped

### Instructions

- At first Season the beef with salt and pepper. Next Toss with flour.
- Then Place the oil in the Instant Pot and turn on to the "Saute" mode. Once the oil is hot, add the beef and brown all on sides, letting the meat caramelize and brown before turning it.
- After that Add the beef broth to the pot and use a wooden spoon to scrape up any bits on the bottom of the pan. Then add the Worcestershire sauce, garlic cloves, bay leaves, salt, sugar, paprika, pepper, and thyme. Stir so that the spices are incorporated into the broth.
- In the next step Add the remaining ingredients and stir. Add the lid and close the steam valve. Press the "meat/stew" button or set the timer to 35 minutes on high pressure. After the 35 minutes, let the pressure release naturally. Once the pressure is released, release the steam valve and open the lid carefully. Season with salt and pepper if needed.
- Slow Cooker: Finally Add everything to the slow cooker and cook on low for 8 hours.

**Nutrition Facts Per Serving** Calories 304 / Calories from Fat 74 / Cholesterol 72mg

# Instant Pot Vegetable Soup

Prep Time 5 mins // Cook Time 25 mins
Serves 6 // **Points Values:1**

## Ingredients

- 2 tsp olive oil & 1 yellow onion, chopped
- 4 garlic cloves, minced & 3/4 tsp dried oregano
- 3/4 tsp dried thyme & 12 oz. Simple Truth Frozen Organic Mixed Vegetables
- 12 oz. Simple Truth Frozen Organic Green Beans & 1 (14 oz.) can petite diced tomatoes
- 2 3/4 cups vegetable broth & 1/2 tsp salt
- 1/2 tsp ground pepper , 1/4 cup chopped flat-leaf parsley & Salt and pepper, to taste

## Instructions

- At first Set Instant Pot to the saute setting. Next Add the olive oil and allow to heat for 1 minute. Then Add the onion and cook, stirring occasionally, until softened, about 5 minutes. Stir in the garlic, oregano and thyme, and cook for 1 minute.
- After that Add the frozen mix vegetables, frozen green beans, petite diced tomatoes, vegetable broth, salt and pepper, and stir to combine.
- In the next step Put the lid on the Instant Pot, close the steam vent and set to HIGH pressure using the manual setting. Decrease the time to 4 minutes.
- Finally Once the time is expired, wait for 5 minutes, then carefully use the quick release valve to release the steam. Stir in the parsley. Season to taste. Serve.

**Nutrition Facts Per Serving** Serving Size 1 1/3 cups / Amount Per Serving As Served / Calories 102.2 cal Calories from fat 9 / Total Fat 1.9g// Saturated Fat 0.3g //Cholesterol 0mg

## Cheesy Turkey Burger Macaroni

Prep Time: 10 mins // Cook Time: 20 mins
Servings: 8 // **Points Values:8**

### *Ingredients*

- 1 Tablespoon olive oil & 1 pound lean ground turkey
- 1 medium onion chopped & 1/2 teaspoon salt
- 1/4 teaspoon black pepper & 1/2 teaspoon dried thyme
- 1/4 cup ketchup & 2 cups elbow macaroni
- 3 cups beef stock & 8 oz Fontina cheese grated

### *Instructions*

- At first Heat the olive oil on SAUTE mode with the pressure cooker's lid off. Next Place the turkey into the cooker and cook until it's browned, about 5 minutes.
- Then Add the remaining ingredients, except for the cheese, to the cooker. Securely lock the lid and set on MANUAL for 6 minutes at HIGH pressure.
- Perform a quick release to release the pressure. Finally Add the shredded Fontina cheese and stir until it's melted and creamy. Serve immediately.

***Nutrition Facts Per Serving*** Calories: 332kcal / Carbohydrates: 24.6g / Protein: 23.3g / Fat: 15.8g // Saturated Fat: 7g //Cholesterol: 74.8mg

| Spicy Asian Chicken Soup |

20 minPrep Time // 25 minCook Time
Servings: 6 // **Points Values:6**

## *Ingredients*

- 2 cups chicken breast, cubed into bite sized pieces & 2 teaspoons coconut oil
- 1/2 cup onion, chopped & 2 cups carrots, shredded
- 8 ounces mushroom, sliced & 6 cups low sodium chicken broth
- 2 teaspoons chili garlic sauce, add more if you like heat & 2 teaspoons ginger, minced
- 1 tablespoon low sodium soy sauce & 14 ounces bean sprouts, canned, rinsed, and drained
- 2 cups brown rice, cooked (optional) , 3/4 cup green onion, sliced & 3/4 cup cilantro, chopped

## *Instructions*

- First Heat the instant pot on the saute mode (or saute in a stock pot over medium-high heat). Next Add coconut oil and allow to get hot. Add chicken and onions and cook for 3 - 5 minutes.
- Then Add carrots and mushrooms and cook another 5 minutes stirring often.
- After that Add broth, chili garlic sauce, ginger, and soy sauce. Turn the Instant Pot to pressure cook mode on high for 10 minutes. Use quick release mode when the timer goes off. If you aren't using an Instant Pot, continue to cook chicken soup over the stove for 25 - 30 minutes until chicken is cooked through and vegetables are softened.
- In the next step Add bean sprouts and rice to the pot and allow to heat through.
- Finally Serve with green onion and cilantro.

**Nutrition Facts Per Serving** Food energy: 252kcal / Saturated fatty acids: 2.29g /Total fat: 4.71g / Calories from fat: 42 /Cholesterol: 55mg / Carbohydrate, by difference: 25.86g

## Chicken Enchilada Soup

Prep Time: 10 mins//Cook Time: 30 mins
Servings : 6 // **Points Values:1**

### *Ingredients*

- 1 lb chicken breasts (skinless, boneless) & 1 tbsp avocado oil
- 1 small onion (diced) & 4 cloves of garlic minced
- 3 cups fat free chicken broth & 15 oz can diced fire roasted tomatoes
- 10 oz can red enchilada sauce & 15 oz can black beans (drained and rinsed)
- 2 cups frozen corn & 1/2 cup cilantro (chopped)
- 1 tbsp canned chipotles in adobo sauce (chopped) & 1 tbsp ground cumin
- Salt and pepper to taste & Juice of 1 lime

### *Instructions*

- First Set Instant Pot to saute. When hot, add in oil. Then add in onions and garlic, and saute until tender, about 2 minutes.
- Then Pour in the chicken broth, enchilada sauce, diced tomatoes, chipotle in adobo sauce, beans, corn, cumin, salt and pepper. Stir well.
- After that Add in chicken breasts, making sure chicken is fully covered with sauce. Cover and cook on high pressure for 20 minutes. Release quick or natural.
- Finally Shred chicken with two forks, and stir in cilantro and lime juice. Taste and adjust seasonings as needed. Spoon into bowls. Garnish as desired and serve.

**Nutrition Facts Per Serving** Calories 231 Calories from Fat 31 / Total Fat 3.4g 5% /Saturated Fat 0.3g 2% /Cholesterol 44mg 15% /Sodium 442mg 18% / Potassium 749mg

# Skinny Steak Soup

Prep Time: 5 mins // Cook Time: 20 mins
Servings: 4 // **Points Values: 3**

## Ingredients

- 1 lb Steak or stew meat, fat trimmed & 1 Onion diced
- 2 Carrots diced
- 2 Celery Stalk diced & 4 sweet peppers diced (or 1 large bell pepper)
- 8 oz mushrooms cremini, button sliced thin & 2 tbsp garlic powder
- 2 tsp celtic sea salt & 2 tsp oregano
- 1 tsp thyme & 1 bay leaf
- 1 cup crushed tomatoes, 2 cups beef stock & 2 cups water

## Instructions

- First Set Instant pot to saute (or heat a large stock pot to medium).
- Next Add stew meat and brown.
- Then Add onion, celery, pepper, carrots, and cook until softened.
- After that Add mushrooms, cook until soft.
- In the next step Add spices, salt, water, and stock and cover instant pot, setting to seal. (or cover with lid and set to low if cooking on stove.)
- Cook on soup setting for 15 minutes (if cooking on stovetop, cook on low for 1 hour).
- Finally Release steam and serve hot.

**Nutrition Facts Per Serving** Calories 364 Calories from Fat 153 / Total Fat 17g / Saturated Fat 7g / Cholesterol 69mg / Sodium 431mg

# Instant Pot Beef and Barley Stew

Prep Time: 10 Min // Cook Time: 45 Min
Serving Size: 1.25-1.5 cups // **Points Values:7**

## Ingredients

- 1.5 lbs lean beef stew meat
- 2 tsp flour
- 2 tsp olive oil
- 1 onion, diced
- 1 cup carrots, diced
- 1 cup celery, diced
- 2 tbsp. tomato paste
- 4 garlic cloves, diced
- 6 cups beef broth
- 2 bay leaves
- 3/4 tsp thyme
- 2/3 cup pearl barley, rinsed
- 2 cups hash brown potatoes

## Instructions

- First Turn the Instant Pot on Saute mode. Next Once hot add the oil. Then Toss the beef with flour, salt, and pepper. Add to the instant pot and brown on both sides, about 5-7 minutes. You may want to do this in two batches to get a more intense flavor since the beef will brown more. Remove the beef and set aside.
- After that Add the onions, celery, and carrots. Cook for 4-5 minutes. Add the tomato paste and garlic. Cook until fragrant, about 1 minute.
- In the next step Add the beef broth, bay leaves, thyme, and pearl barley. Stir together.
- Close the Instant Pot and press the Soup/Stew button and set for 25 minutes. Let pressure release naturally once finished cooking. Open and add the potatoes. Let cook for 5 minutes until potatoes warm up. Season with salt and pepper.

- Finally Slow Cooker Option: Follow steps 1 and 2 using a large pan. Add those ingredients to the slow cooker along with the broth, bay leaves, thyme, and barley. Cook on low for 8 hours. Stir in the potatoes and let cook for 10 minutes more or until potatoes are warmed through. Season with salt and pepper.

**Nutrition Facts Per Serving** Calories 329 //Calories from Fat 70

# Beef and Tomato Stew

Prep Time: 20 Min // Cook Time: 23 Min
Serves: 8 // **Points Values:6**

## *Ingredients*

- 1 Tbsp olive oil (if searing the meat first) & 2 lb. cubed stew beef
- 1 (15 oz) can stewed tomatoes & 1 (6 oz) can tomato paste
- 2 cups beef broth & 1 Tbsp Worcestershire sauce
- 1 medium onion, chopped & 3 large carrots, sliced
- 3 ribs celery, chopped & 1 cup fresh or frozen peas
- 1 lb. baby potatoes & 1 tsp. salt & ½ tsp. pepper
- 2 tsp. garlic powder , 1 Tbsp fresh thyme (or 1 tsp dried) & 2 tsp fresh rosemary (or ½ tsp dried) & 1 bay leaf

## *Instructions*

- To make in your instant pot: First Drizzle olive oil in the bowl of your instant pot and turn on the sauté function. Next Wait until it's nice and heated then add meat, browning on all sides. Then Add the rest of your ingredients, seal the instant pot and select the meat/stew setting (about 35 minutes). Once cooking is complete, let the instant pot sit for about 12 minutes then release the steam by placing the valve to the venting position.
- To make in your slow cooker: Add cubed beef (except the oil) along with the rest of ingredients, cover and cook on low for 7 to 8 hours.
- To make on your stove top: Finally In a large dutch oven or pot on medium high heat, drizzle oil and sear meat on all sides. Add the rest of the ingredients and bring to a boil, then cover and simmer for about 2 to 3 hours, until meat is tender. Serve and enjoy!

**Nutrition Facts Per Serving** Serving Size: 1½ cups /Calories: 325 /Fat: 13.3 g

# Chicken Curry Recipe with Potatoes

Prep Time 10 mins// Cook Time 25 mins
Serves 6 // **Points Values:9**

## Ingredients

- 2 tsp olive oil , 1/2 yellow onion, chopped & 1/2 Gala apple, chopped , 2 tbsp minced ginger
- 4 garlic cloves, minced & 6 tbsp mild curry paste
- 2 tsp ground coriander & 2 tsp ground cumin
- 2 tsp garam masala & 2 lb. boneless, skinless chicken thighs
- 1 lb. Little Potato Company Creamer potatoes (halved or quartered)* & 1 1/2 cup diced tomatoes
- 3/4 cup chicken broth & 3/4 cuplite coconut milk & 1/2 tsp salt & 1/2 tsp ground pepper

## Instructions

- First Set the Instant Pot to the saute setting. Next Add the olive oil and allow to heat for 1 minute. Then Add the onion, apple and ginger, and cook, stirring occasionally, until softened, about 5 minutes. Stir in the garlic, curry paste, coriander, cumin and garam masala, and cook for 1 minute.
- After that Add the chicken thighs, potatoes, tomatoes, chicken broth, coconut milk, salt and pepper, and stir to combine.
- Put the lid on the Instant Pot, close the steam vent and set to HIGH pressure using the manual setting. Decrease the time to 10 minutes.
- Finally Once the time is expired, wait for 5 minutes, then carefully use the quick release valve to release the steam. Shred the chicken with two forks. Season to taste. Serve.

**Nutrition Facts Per Serving** Serving Size 1 cup / Calories 349.8 cal /Calories from fat 144

# Chicken and Dumplings

Serves: 6 servings // **Points Values:5**

## Ingredients

- 1 cup frozen corn & 1 cup carrots, chopped or sliced
- 3-4 stalks celery, chopped & 5 cups (99% fat free) chicken broth
- 1 pound boneless, skinless chicken breasts & 2 cups Bisquick Original Pancake and Baking Mix
- 1 cup fat-free milk & 1 cup frozen peas, optional
- Fresh snipped parsley, optional & Salt and pepper, to taste

## Instructions

- At first Add corn, carrots, and celery to the Instant Pot. Pour chicken broth over the vegetables.
- Next Carefully add chicken to the Instant pot. Set IP to HIGH and set to cook for 10 minutes if chicken is frozen and 8 minutes if the chicken is thawed.
- Meanwhile, in a small bowl, mix Bisquick with milk and set aside.
- In the next stepQuick release after the 10 minutes cooking time is up, to let the pressure out. Take the lid off, but keep the IP on HIGH heat. Take chicken out of the IP and shred the chicken with two forks.
- (Add peas to the IP if you will be using them) Add chicken back to the IP being careful not to splatter hot broth up onto your hands and being mindful of the sides of the IP that will be hot.
- Carefully add 1 tablespoon scoops of the Bisquick mixture into the hot broth and allow to cook until the dumplings are no longer dough-like, about 8-10 minutes, flipping over the dumplings about half-way through cooking time.
- Finally Turn off heat on the IP and served. Salt and pepper to taste. Top with optional parsley if you will be using it.

**Nutrition Facts Per Serving** Serving size: 1-2/3 c. soup & 4 dumplings / Calories: 276 / Fat: 5 g /Saturated fat: 1 g / Trans fat: 0 g /Carbohydrates: 38 g /Cholesterol: 38 mg

# Chicken and Rice Recipe

Prep Time 10 mins// Cook Time 40 mins
Servings: 6 // Serving size is about 1 ¼ cups // **Points Values:6**

## Ingredients

- 1 ½ lbs chicken thighs (skinless, boneless) & 1 cup brown rice (uncooked and rinsed)
- 1 tbsp olive oil & 2 ¼ cup fat free chicken broth
- 1 large onion (finely chopped) & 2 large carrots (diced)
- 8 oz mushrooms (sliced) & 4 cloves garlic (minced)
- 2 tsp dried thyme , 1 tbsp fresh lemon juice & Salt and pepper to taste

## Instructions

- At first Turn Instant Pot to "Saute". When hot, add olive oil.
- Next Season chicken with salt and pepper, then in the chicken, and brown about 3-4 minutes on each side. Remove chicken and set aside.
- Then Deglaze the pot by pouring in ¼ cup of the chicken broth, and making sure to scrape up the browned bits on the bottom of the pan.
- After that Add in all the chopped vegetables, and saute for about 3 minutes.
- In the next stepStir in the remaining broth, thyme, lemon juice and rice. Add additional salt and pepper as desired. Top with the chicken.
- Turn off the "Saute" function. Lock on lid, select the "Manual" function and set to high pressure for 20 minutes.
- Finally Allow to naturally release for 10 minutes, then manually release any remaining pressure. Transfer chicken to plates and serve!

**Nutrition Facts Per Serving** Calories 345 Calories from Fat 90 / Total Fat 10g / Saturated Fat 2.4g / Cholesterol 93mg / Sodium 419mg / Potassium 410mg

## Buffalo Chicken Lettuce Wraps

Prep Time:5 mins// Cook Time:4 hours
Servings:6, Serving Size: 1/2 cup + veggies // **Points Values:0**

*Ingredients:*
For the chicken:

- 24 oz (3) boneless skinless chicken breasts & 1 celery stalk
- 1/2 onion, diced & 1 clove garlic
- 16 oz fat free low sodium chicken broth & 1/2 cup cayenne pepper sauce (I used Frank's)

For the wraps:
- 6 large lettuce leaves, Bibb or Iceberg
- 1 1/2 cups shredded carrots
- 2 large celery stalks, cut into 2 inch matchsticks

*Instructions*

- First Combine chicken, onions, celery stalk, garlic and broth (enough to cover your chicken, use water if the can of broth isn't enough) in the Instant Pot. Next Cover and cook high pressure 15 minutes. Natural release.
- Then Remove the chicken from pot, reserve 1/2 cup broth and discard the rest. Shred the chicken with two forks, return to the pot with the 1/2 cup broth and the hot sauce and saute 2 to 3 minutes. Makes 3 cups chicken.
- Finally To prepare lettuce cups, place 1/2 cup buffalo chicken in each leaf, top with 1/4 cup shredded carrots, celery and dressing of your choice. Wrap up and start eating!

**Nutrition Facts Per Serving** Calories: 147.5 calories// Total Fat: 0.1g / Saturated Fat: g / Cholesterol: mg

# Instant Pot Chicken Soup

Prep Time15 mins, Cook Time 30 mins
Servings:12 // **Points Values:9**

## *Ingredients*

- 2 tbsp olive oil & 2 cups yellow onion (chopped)
- 2 tsp minced garlic & 1 cup celery (chopped)
- 1 tbsp turmeric & 1 tbsp Italian seasoning
- 2 tsp ground black pepper & 2 tsp salt (or to taste)
- 1 whole chicken (3-4 lbs) & 2 cups cut carrots
- 3 cups baby red potatoes (quartered) & 4 cups chicken broth

## *Instructions*

- First Set the Instant Pot to Saute and let warm.
- Next Add olive oil.
- Then Once olive oil is warm, add chopped onion and saute for 2 to 3 minutes continually stirring.
- After that Add minced garlic and cook for another 1 to 2 minutes. Continue to stir.
- In the next stepStir in chopped celery.
- Meanwhile Add turmeric, Italian seasoning, pepper and salt. Mix all the ingredients well and let saute for an additional 1 to 2 minutes.
- Place whole chicken, breast side up, into the Instant Pot.
- Add the carrots, baby red potatoes and chicken broth.
- Turn the Instant Pot off and then close the lid.
- Ensure that the pressure release handle is set to sealing.
- Select the Soup function on your Instant Pot. The Instant Pot will cook at high pressure for 30 minutes.
- Once the Instant Pot has completed cooking, allow for a full natural pressure release (NPR).
- Ensure that all pressure has been released before opening the pot.
- Carefully remove the whole chicken from the Instant Pot and place in a bowl and shred. Add the shredded chicken back to your soup.
- Finally Your chicken soup is ready to serve!

**Nutrition Facts Per Serving** Calories 215 Calories from Fat 36 / Total Fat 4g 6% / Cholesterol 108mg 36% / Sodium 521mg 22% / Potassium 786mg 22% / Total Carbohydrates 4g

## Brussels Sprouts with Bacon and Garlic

Prep Time 5 mins // Cook Time 15 mins
Servings 4 // **Points Values:1**

### *Ingredients*

- 1 pound fresh Brussels Sprouts & 3 cloves garlic minced
- 3 shallots diced fine , 4 slices center cut bacon cut into 1/2" pieces & 1/2 cup water

### *Instructions*

- First Prepare Brussels sprouts by removing stems and halving larger pieces so they become bite-sized.
- Next Mince garlic cloves, slice shallots and cut bacon into small pieces.
- Then Turn Instant Pot to Saute, and add bacon to Instant Pot liner. Cook for 5-7 minutes or until it begins to render and crisp.
- After that Add the remaining ingredients and stir well.
- In the next step Place lid on Instant Pot and set to seal.
- Cook on manual high pressure for 4 minutes.
- Finally Quick release and serve.

**Nutrition Facts Per Serving** Amount Per Serving (4 oz) / Calories 194 Calories from Fat 117 / Total Fat 13g 20% / Saturated Fat 4g 20% / Cholesterol 21mg 7% / Sodium 538mg 2

## Meatloaf Mashed Potatoes

Prep Time: 10 mins // Cook Time: 35 mins
Serving Size: 6 // **Points Values:11**

***Ingredients*** -For the Meatloaf:
- 2 lb. ground beef (I used a lean ground beef) & 1 cup breadcrumbs
- 2 eggs & 1/2 cup onion, diced
- 2 tsp garlic powder & 2 tsp dried parsley
- 1 tsp salt and pepper& 1/2 cup honey bbq sauce

For the Meatloaf Topping:
- 2 tbsp brown sugar
- 2 tbsp mustard
- 1/3 cup ketchup

For the potatoes:
- 3 lbs. yellow potatoes, washed and quartered & 1 cup chicken broth
- 1 cup half and half & 4 tbsp butter
- 3/4 cup sour cream, 1 tsp garlic powder & salt and pepper to taste

***Instructions***

- First Start by laying the quartered potatoes in the bottom of your pressure cooker in an even layer. Next Pour the chicken broth over the top. Then Lay the rack that comes with your pressure cooker over the top so it lays flat.
- After that Combine the ingredients for the meatloaf (minus the topping) in a large bowl until fully combined. Shape the meat mixture into a loaf and place on a piece of tinfoil. Shape the tinfoil up and around the edges of the meatloaf, creating a pocket for it. Place the meatloaf on top of the rack in the pressure cooker and secure lid.

- Ensure that the steam release is closed and turn pressure cooker to Manual mode for 20 to 25 minutes*. Once finished cooking, use the quick release method to let the steam escape. Check meatloaf for internal temperature of 155 degrees.
- Carefully lift the meatloaf out of the pressure cooker and place on a baking sheet. Mix the ingredients for the topping and brush all over the meatloaf. Place meatloaf under the broiler for just 3 to 4 minutes, until the top is bubbly and caramelized.
- Meanwhile add the remaining ingredients (half and half, butter, sour cream, garlic powder, salt and pepper) to the instant pot and mash the potatoes until smooth and creamy.
- Finally Serve the meatloaf in slices with the mashed potatoes. Enjoy!

# Mushroom Barley Soup

Prep Time 10 mins // Cook Time 30 mins
Servings 8 , Serving size is 1 1/2 cups // **Points Values:2**

## Ingredients

- 8 cups beef broth & 3/4 cup barley
- one medium onion chopped & 2 carrots chopped
- 4 cloves garlic minced & 1 lb sliced mushrooms
- 1 tsp salt , 1/2 tsp freshly ground pepper & 1 Tbsp Steak Sauce

## Instructions

- First Add all ingredients to the Instant Pot and stir well.
- Next Set Instant Pot to Manual / High Pressure for 20 minutes.
- Then Let pressure release naturally for 10 minutes then Quick Release
- Finally Stir well & Enjoy!

**Nutrition Facts Per Serving** Amount Per Serving (1 g)

# Light Stuffed Pepper Soup

Prep Time 20 mins // Cook Time 8 hrs
Servings: 8 // **Points Values:2**

## Ingredients

- 1 lb extra lean ground turkey or beef & 1 cup onion chopped
- 14.5 oz. can diced tomatoes with roasted garlic and onions & 15 oz. can tomato sauce
- 2 cups green and red peppers chopped (I've added up to four peppers, and it's yummy!) & 3 cups beef broth
- ½ teaspoon basil, 1.5 packets of chili seasoning & 1 cup cooked rice brown or white

## Instructions

- At first Brown ground beef with onion in a skillet over medium heat.
- Next Drain beef and onions and place in crock pot.
- Then Chop peppers, add to crock pot.
- After that Add tomatoes (including juice) and remaining ingredients, except rice – which should be added 1 hour before end of cooking.
- Finally Cover and cook on low for 6-8 hours.

**Notes :** Instant Pot Adaptation: Saute the meat and onion, then add peppers, tomatoes and tomato sauce, broth, and spices. Cook at high pressure 7 minutes, add cooked rice after. For Weight Watchers this is 2 Freestyle Smart Points per serving when using lean ground turkey!

**Nutrition Facts Per Serving** Calories: 247kcal

| # Boneless Pork Chops Recipe |
|---|

[Prep Time :5 mins] [Cook Time :5 mins] [ Pressure Release :10 mins] [Total Time :10 mins]

Servings: 6 // **Points Values:3**

## Ingredients

- 1 tablespoon coconut oil & 4-6 boneless pork chops
- 1 stick of butter or margarine , 1 package of ranch mix & 1 cup water

## Instructions

- At first Place the pork chops in the Instant pot with a tablespoon of coconut oil. Next Turn on the saute setting and brown on both sides. Then Make sure all pork chops are browned. You can skip this step but they look prettier when you brown them first.
- After that Place the butter on top and sprinkle the ranch mix packet on top.
- In the next stepPour water (or chicken broth) over the pork.
- Place the lid on and set to sealing.
- Push the manual button and set to 5 minutes.
- Allow it to naturally release pressure for 5 minutes and then do a quick release to remove the rest of the pressure.
- Once cooked, serve.
- Finally You can even spoon the buttery sauce over the pork chops and over your veggies when serving.

**Nutrition Facts Per Serving** Calories 372 Calories from Fat 207 / Total Fat 23g 35% //Saturated Fat 13g 65% //Cholesterol 152mg 51% // Sodium 233mg 10% //Potassium 658mg 19% //Protein 38g

www.ingramcontent.com/pod-product-compliance
Lightning Source LLC
Chambersburg PA
CBHW050115230526
45470CB00004B/1848